23.95

# HOMICIDAL INSANITY, 1800–1985

## History of American Science and Technology Series

### General Editor, LESTER D. STEPHENS

*The Eagle's Nest: Natural History and American Ideas, 1812–1842*
by Charlotte M. Porter

*Nathaniel Southgate Shaler and the Culture of American Science*
by David N. Livingstone

*Henry William Ravenel, 1814–1887: South Carolina Scientist in the Civil War Era*
by Tamara Miner Haygood

*Granville Sharp Pattison: Anatomist and Antagonist, 1781–1851*
by Frederick L. M. Pattison

*Making Medical Doctors: Science and Medicine at Vanderbilt since Flexner*
by Timothy C. Jacobson

*U.S. Coast Survey vs. Naval Hydrographic Office: A 19th-Century Rivalry in Science and Politics*
by Thomas G. Manning

*Homicidal Insanity, 1800–1985*
by Janet Colaizzi

# HOMICIDAL INSANITY, 1800–1985

JANET COLAIZZI

Foreword by Jonas R. Rappeport

The University of Alabama Press

Tuscaloosa and London

Library of Congress Cataloging-in-Publication
Data
Colaizzi, Janet, 1936–
    Homicidal insanity, 1800–1985.

    (History of American science and technology
series)
    Bibliography: p.
    Includes index.
    1. Forensic psychiatry—History.   2. Homicide—
Psychological aspects.   3. Insane, Criminal and
dangerous.   I. Title.   II. Series.   [DNLM: 1.
Forensic Psychiatry—history.   2. Homicide—
history.   3. Mental Disorders—history.   WM
11.1 C683h]
RA1151.C8   1989      614.1      88-1154
ISBN 0-8173-0404-5 (alk. paper)

British Library Cataloguing-in-Publication Data
                          available

# Contents

# Foreword

The last week of 1987 produced three mass murders. *Russelville, Arkansas.* R. Gene Simmons, Sr., killed sixteen people. "I've gotten everybody who wanted to hurt me," a witness heard him say. Shortly before he surrendered, he told a hostage, "I've come to do what I wanted to do. It's all over now." *Algona, Iowa.* "Seven family members were found shot to death . . . in what may have been a murder-suicide. . . . Police said Robert Dreesman, 40, shot his parents, his sister, and her three children with his shotgun before taking his own life." *Nashua, New Hampshire.* "A man with a history of drug charges went on a shooting rampage in two communities, killing three men and critically wounding two before police shot him dead, authorities said yesterday. . . . All told, fifty-two relatives of killers were slain in eight mass murders in 1987, which sociologists say is the highest number of family massacres in recent memory."

In the three year-end mass murders we will have the opportunity to evaluate only one of the perpetrators. Psychological autopsies may give us some insight into the minds of two of the murderers. However, those will not be as complete as the full psychiatric evaluation which Mr. Simmons will undergo. Undoubtedly he will enter an insanity plea. There will be a "battle of the experts." It would be unusual if a number of psychiatric experts did not express varying opinions about his sanity. This is nothing new, as Dr. Colaizzi has made clear in her excellent volume on the history of homicidal insanity. She points out that even in 1840, "differences of theoretical opinion surfaced in medico-legal cases in which alienists publicly disagreed."

In my thirty years in forensic psychiatry, I have come to accept the disagreement among experts. After all, opposing attorneys would not call upon experts if they did not disagree. We never hear about cases in which the experts agree, because these trials are abbreviated by the prosecutor who recommends that the court accept the plea of insanity. What was intriguing to me in reading this book was the fact that ever since there have been experts, there has been disagreement among them. They used to ask: Was the moral faculty impaired? Was the intelligence inadequate? Were there delusions? The "cult of delusions" appears to be as old as the insanity plea itself. Today's theories only produce different questions.

In the Hinckley case, which led to the public's current interest in the insanity plea, the prosecution's psychiatrists did not believe John Hinckley, Jr., was delusional, while the defense's experts believed he was. The jury agreed with the defense and found him not guilty by reason of insanity. These disagreements have preoccupied us since ancient times. Over centuries the legal test has changed, as has our knowledge of the human mind. Neither the law nor medical science is perfect, so we should expect both change and disagreement. What is sobering is the fact that no matter what theoretical constructs are promulgated, they are certain to change within fifty to one hundred years. Also sobering is the fact that the new theories are no better at answering the legal question of insanity than those of the past.

Unfortunately for psychiatry, our problems do not end when a person is declared "not guilty by reason of insanity" or, as some jurisdictions currently name the plea, "guilty but not responsible because of mental disorder." Colaizzi does not stop there either. What is to be done with the acquittee after such a finding? Things were easier in the days of Daniel M'Naghten; he was committed to the hospital for life and died there. Today we must struggle with the issue of discharge when the patient is no longer dangerous. When is it safe to release a "homicidal maniac" into the community? In 1845, Beck, speaking of monomaniacs, agreed that "one who has been guilty of a heinous crime like murder should never, on any pretense, be discharged." Today, discharge decisions must be based on a thorough psychiatric evaluation and, where required, judicial decision. Colaizzi discusses the changes that have occurred in our evaluation of dangerousness and society's tolerance of mental illness over the almost two hundred years covered by her treatise.

I recently chaired a subcommittee of the American Psychiatric Association's Council on Psychiatry and the Law that was charged to review the APA's 1982 statement on the insanity plea. The subcommittee could not find clear evidence that harm had resulted from the APA's recommendation for the elimination of the volitional prong, though some committee members were sure that harm had occurred. Therefore, there was disagreement about whether or not to recommend including the volitional prong in the American Law Institute's version of the insanity plea. There was, however, full agreement among the subcommittee's members that we must involve others—the judiciary, a special board, etc.—in making discharge decisions of insanity acquittees. We agreed that outright discharge should occur only after a substantial period of conditional release. This shared responsibility between psychiatry and the community is long overdue, as one discovers upon reading the problems of the past. As H. G. Wells said, "The past is but the beginning, and all that is and has been is but the twilight of the dawn."

A hundred years ago patients sued for false commitment. Today, patients still sue unless there is a judicial review of the commitment, and we clinicians suffer the pain of the Tarasoff arrows when we fail to restrain or warn of the dangerous patient. The role of the alienist was only slightly easier than that of the modern psychiatrist—easier because there was less accountability. However, while today many of us complain because of so much accountability, we know that there were injustices in those days of yore. Although most of us wish we were less "belegaled" in these days of increased accountability, we know that the law also offers us some protection. Nevertheless, the law, as a representative of society, has never understood much of what psychiatrists talk about, regardless of our theories, when it comes to homicidal insanity. Whether the testimony is from Isaac Ray or from some modern-day forensic giant, the jury must make a social-legal decision. Whether we speak of monomania or schizophrenia, mania transitoria or brief reactive psychosis, moral insanity or antisocial personality, the judge or jury will determine the issue.

Colaizzi has presented a thorough and complete overview of homicidal insanity by the leading alienists—forensic psychiatrists—over a period of 185 years. She has chronicled the theories of the psychiatric community over the past century and a half, but she has also touched on their views of the need for hospitalization, possible discharge, and dangerousness of both the homicidal individual and the seriously mentally ill. She has interwoven the general socio-legal attitudes extant from time to time as they affected the attitudes of psychiatrists. Today we are in yet another phase of what I am confident will be a long, repetitive history of change in our theories, attitudes, and testimony. We will have forever to study and to try to understand, as homicide will surely be forever with us. Those of us who study the mind will just as surely be called upon to try to explain to the court and society why homicide happened.

—Jonas R. Rappeport, M.D.

HOMICIDAL INSANITY, 1800–1985

# The Issue of Insane Homicide

Early in the 1980s, a person who had been under psychiatric care attempted to assassinate the president of the United States. The mass media used this occasion to raise the question of why psychiatrists permitted disturbed and dangerous patients like John Hinckley to move freely in society. The expectation that doctors could and should restrain dangerous lunatics has deep roots in the past. The consequent professional dilemma emerged not only in the case of John Hinckley but also throughout the history of psychiatry.

That some mentally ill persons kill is well documented from ancient times to the present. But murder is far from rare, and most murders are not committed by lunatics. Even before there were any medical specialists in mental diseases, a physician was often summoned to decide whether or not a mad person was dangerous.

This book is about homicidal insanity. Its purpose is to describe how physicians have diagnosed, explained, and restrained the dangerous insane from the beginning of medical care for the mentally ill to the present. The issue of homicidal insanity is embedded in the scientific and social history of medicine on the Continent and in the United States; and, despite the panorama of change over a 200-year span, it has remained a central social issue and a conundrum for psychiatry.

3

From the beginning, it was clear that some lunatics were harmless and some were dangerous. Psychiatrists had to find ways to diagnose homicidal insanity. Early medical writers on insanity, notably Philippe Pinel in France and Benjamin Rush in the United States, instructed their readers on the differential diagnosis and management of dangerous lunatics. As the literature of insanity grew, European, British, and American writers recounted celebrated cases of insane homicide and contributed their own clinical experience. Throughout nearly 200 years of Anglo-American psychiatry, cases of insane homicide were reported that were clinically similar, generation after generation. Although the nosology was inconsistent and subject to debate and controversy, the mental phenomena these early clinicians identified as evidence of homicidal insanity were the same.

The predominant opinion today among psychiatrists is that no correlation exists between dangerousness and specific mental disorders. Research published in the last two decades has failed to demonstrate any positive correlation between mental illness and criminal offenses.[1] Although psychiatrists have not found a correlation between insane homicide and any disorders classified in the *Diagnostic and Statistical Manual III*, the current literature reflects the belief that specific mental phenomena are predictors of dangerousness when the patient's social situation is taken into account.

The organizing principle of the nosology during the early decades of the nineteenth century was faculty psychology. Psychiatrists focused upon the manifestations of the disease and subdivided insanity into derangements of the intellect, the emotions, and the will.[2] Later in the century, medical science developed organ and cellular pathology. But psychiatry had no such science.

### Theories of Homicidal Insanity

Scientific, intellectual, and social changes influenced the way in which psychiatrists explained insanity. Throughout the nineteenth century, they agreed that it was disease of the brain. Some theorists conceived of localized brain functions and suggested that homicidal insanity could be traced to the pathology of specific cortical structures. But the examination techniques of the times failed to reveal any differences between the brains of homicidal lunatics and harmless lunatics; and, except for brain tumors and vascular disorders, between the brains of the insane and the sane. Later psychiatrists maintained the somatic model, but believed that insanity was a diffuse rather than a localized cortical disease. Lacking a specific brain pathology, they continued to think in terms of a phenomenology of insanity.

Most nineteenth-century psychiatrists believed that the brain was affected by outside forces or by any organ of the body. Knowledge of the pathways and mechanisms through which these influences reached the brain changed with an evolving medical science. Still, situational and physiological forces could derange the brain and cause insanity. It followed logically that intense forces could produce homicidal insanity.

With the rise of psychoanalytic concepts, some psychiatrists posited dynamic explanations for insane homicide. This theoretical excursus did not displace the predominant somatic model. In both models, however, interest in the hereditarian and constitutional origins of dangerous insanity has continued throughout two centuries.

## Involuntary Commitment and Restraint

Psychiatrists applied their theoretical knowledge and belief to the practical matters of prediction and prevention. At first, the predominant issues were the management of homicidal lunatics in the asylum and the question of when to turn them loose. Not all asylum superintendents had the legal authority to discharge patients, but generally this decision was their responsibility and they were morally, if not legally, responsible for any harm caused by a former patient.[3]

Involuntary commitment to an asylum was not restricted to the homicidal insane. The belief that the mentally ill, whether dangerous or harmless, should be restrained for their own good is firmly rooted in Anglo-American law. Throughout the nineteenth and well into the twentieth century, psychiatrists and social thinkers regarded the mentally ill as absolutely incompetent and subject to the guardianship of the state. Dorothea Dix, the nineteenth-century reformer of psychiatric care, argued that the state is responsible for providing care to these helpless insane. The doctrine of *parens patriae*, that the state should relate to its citizens as a parent to the child, was the basis for involuntary institutionalization of all the mentally ill.

Social thinkers challenged *parens patriae* from time to time, but is has only been since the social changes of the 1960s that the criterion of dangerousness has predominated in psychiatric and legal thinking. Civil libertarian thinkers believed that no amount of humanitarian concern was sufficient to deprive citizens of their liberty. Although this belief has influenced involuntary commitment from time to time over the past 200 years, it has only been since the 1960s that increased attention to the standard of dangerousness has led to revision of commitment statutes in most states. More and more, the sole criterion for involuntary commitment is becoming this standard. Yet, since 1974, the official position of the American Psychiatric Association has been that it cannot be predicted.[4]

### Insanity and Crime

Early in the development of the specialty, psychiatrists were called upon by the legal system to defend the irresponsible and to expose the culpable. Both medical and legal experts searched for the elusive test for insanity. Substantial controversy within both the medical and the legal professions has honed the essential questions, but no rational method exists to this day to discriminate insanity from crime.

Theoretical formulations directly affected the methods psychiatrists used to separate the insane from the criminal. Religious ideas about the brain/mind relationship collided with problems of free will and responsibility. Most psychiatrists adopted the tenets of the Scottish common-sense school, which balanced the objective physical reality of human existence with theoretical concepts about innate moral faculties. The philosophical and scientific dilemmas of both psychiatry and the law have been no more evident than in the courts.

### Phenomenology of Homicidal Insanity

The central thesis of this book is that, from the beginning, psychiatrists have associated homicidal insanity with certain psychiatric phenomena. The term phenomenon is used in this context because, as theory changed, practitioners regarded such events variously as symptoms of mental disease or the disease itself. Further, some theorists regarded a particular phenomenon as pathological, but others regarded it as insignificant or denied its existence altogether. Some psychiatrists believed that the appearance of these phenomena in a particular patient clearly made that person dangerous. It is possible to trace these phenomena throughout 200 years of Anglo-American psychiatric theory and practice (figure 1). These phenomena are: (1) delusions; (2) command hallucinations (Intellectual Insanity); (3) lack of remorse, or "moral feelings"; (4) morbid impulses (Emotional Insanity); and (5) mania, or "frenzy" (Volitional Insanity).

A secondary thesis is that psychiatrists have used these predictors in the practical matter of preventing insane homicide. Notwithstanding the philosophical, scientific, social, and legal vexations involved, practitioners are clearly responsible for the dangerous insane. In many instances throughout history, they have been given this responsibility with an attenuated authority or with no authority altogether. Still, they were and still are expected to know the difference between the dangerous and harmless insane so that both insane homicide and unwarranted involuntary commitment to mental hospitals can be prevented.

Although the narrative in this volume focuses upon Anglo-American physicians, psychiatry as a medical specialty began in eighteenth-century Europe with the social and scientific changes of the Enlightenment. Early nineteenth-century Anglo-American physicians who were seeking to reform the care of the insane

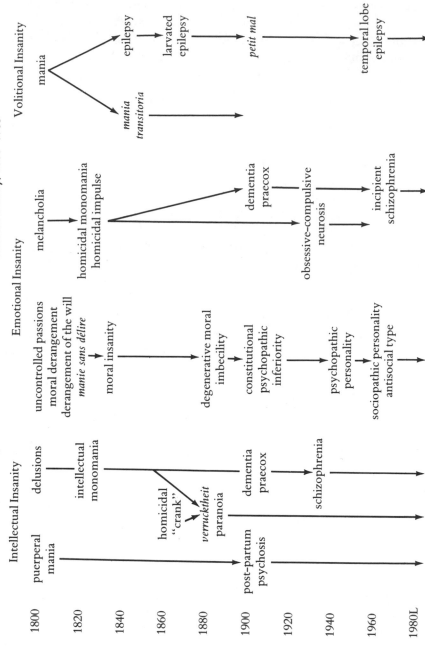

Figure 1. Psychiatric Phenomena Associated with Homicidal Insanity, 1800–1985

looked to European medical authority. To understand how these physicians rationalized their reforms, it is necessary to describe how European ideas were transferred and intertwined through a growing body of clinical experience with the insane.

The story begins at the end of the eighteenth century when the theoretical constructs and lessons learned from contacts with insane patients coalesced into the first medical writings on the subject. Anglo-American physicians took these European ideas, added to them, and formulated their own principles, methods, and techniques. The establishment of asylums and hospitals for the insane institutionalized these reforms.

During the early decades of the nineteenth century, both American and British psychiatrists addressed the jurisprudence of insanity. Throughout the entire history of psychiatry, legal issues commanded the profession's attention. The question of responsibility and justice in insane homicide is a major theme throughout this book.

Psychiatrists have confronted the problem of homicidal insanity in a number of scientific and social contexts. The following chapters trace the intellectual and social changes in the United States and Great Britain over the nineteenth and twentieth centuries and show how they affected psychiatric theory as well as practice in general and particularly in relation to homicidal insanity.

# 2
## The Theoretical Boundaries of Dangerousness 1800–1840

In the United States during the last decades of the eighteenth century, the idea that lunatics should be given medical care in asylums evolved from a number of social and intellectual changes. Among the several changes that guided this transition from family and community care to medical and institutional care, the most evident was the mere fact of population: more lunatics needed to be reckoned with in the growing colonial towns. And, because transients were among the group, the usual practice of family isolation became inapplicable.[1] In complex social groups working together toward common goals, even the merely disruptive are apt to be regarded as dangerous.

The royal governor of Virginia, Francis Fauquier, called for a mental hospital in 1766 and again in 1767. In 1766 his brief message to the opening session of the House of Burgesses reflected Enlightenment beliefs about insanity as the loss of reason, the desire for order in the community, and the idea that the care of the insane was the responsibility of physicians. According to Norman Dain, the real impetus for the hospital project came from an editorial in the *Virginia Gazette*:

A most shocking murder was perpetrated yesterday morning on the body of Mr. Charles Thompson, who lived a little distance from York, by his wife, who for some years past has been out of her senses. He got up early in the morning and walked over his plantation, and when he came home lay down, being much troubled with the headache. He had no sooner got into a doze than his wife came, and with a broadaxe broke his scull to pieces, by repeated strokes. He has left a large family of help-less children. The woman is secured, but seems quite insensible of the horridness of the crime she has committed. (*It is really shocking to see the number of miserable people who have lost the use of their reason, that are daily wandering about, for want of a proper house to keep them confined in. If there had been such a place, this poor man would not have met with the above untimely end.*)[2]

Undoubtedly, as in Virginia, the reform spirit also played a role elsewhere in the shift from family to medical care. Medical and social historians place the genesis of insane asylums squarely within the Enlightenment and post-Enlightenment ideology, which included the concept that even the less fortunate members of society had and could achieve their natural rights. The intel-lectual changes of the Enlightenment, followed by the scientific interest in emotional life, supported the sentimental humanitari-anism that catalyzed the institutional approach. The humanitari-anism that arose during the later Colonial period was rooted in the theory of environmentalism and the idea of progress, that it was within the capacity of man to improve his individual and so-cial conditions.[3]

By the beginning of the nineteenth century, American physi-cians were largely apprentice-trained and gained only a minimum of theoretical knowledge. By this time, however, hospitals were growing in number and size, particularly in Europe, and the con-centration of large numbers of patients in one place provided data for the study of medicine. Physicians were turning to clinical ex-perience as a source of knowledge and began questioning the value of the standard therapeutics that had been handed down virtually unchanged from physician to apprentice for generations. This change was particularly notable in France, where new techniques and new instruments, such as the stethoscope, for example, turned physical diagnosis into a clinical discipline.

By 1820 the French clinical school had begun to have a direct impact upon physicians in the eastern United States, where asylums for the insane were already being established. Under the influence of French clinical empiricism, first on the Continent and then in Great Britain and the United States, physicians began to believe that insanity was a somatic disease and therefore curable. This thesis was reinforced by A. L. J. Bayle's discovery that the symptoms of certain types of insanity could be traced to a definable pathological finding: a chronic inflammation of the brain membrane.[4]

The growth of medical care for the insane in the United States and Great Britain faithfully reflected Continental advances. Even before American physicians began to flock to Paris to study at the large French clinics, William Tuke in England and Benjamin Rush in Philadelphia had already begun clinical treatment of the insane. Moral treatment, an outgrowth of the Enlightenment spirit of humanitarianism, formed a part of the therapeutics, but Rush and his followers also believed that insanity was a somatic disorder and they emphasized medical therapy.

The impetus for American medical interest in the subject, however, came principally from the practical realities of general practice in growing communities. Except for Benjamin Rush and George Parkman, early writers on insanity had no experience in asylum care when their first works were published. Their interest was a response to perceived social need to care for and to protect their charges from injustice. Parkman, for example, in his proposal for the establishment of a retreat for the insane, declared in 1814: "The patient will be courteously received at the Retreat, as a stranger, and he shall not discover that his misfortune is known there, until maniacal extravagance demands his restraint."[5]

Up until the early 1800s, the task of identifying dangerous lunatics did not require any special expertise. But, as the medical profession appropriated responsibility in the field, the task became more complex because clinical observers were identifying not just insanity but its subtle forms.

## The Problem of Homicidal Insanity

Within this context, physicians observed that some lunatics were dangerous and some were not and sought to describe and name the homicidal insanities as well as to differentiate them from the harmless types. From the beginning of this new phase of embryonic psychiatry, the fundamental question of the lunatic's potential dangerousness pervaded the discussions of classification of mental disorders and differential diagnosis.

Physicians observed particularly that homicidal insanity could take different forms. This observation fitted logically into the predominant conception of the mind during the early nineteenth century, a synthesis derived from the rationalist philosophers of the eighteenth century and the Scottish common-sense school. The rationalists posited the mind as separate from the body and possessing three essential functions: (1) reason, or understanding, by which humans perceived and actively synthesized ideas out of experience; (2) the passions, or emotions, by which humans comprehended the feelings; and (3) volition, or will, which gave power to act (or not to act) upon thoughts and feelings. Although philosophers and theologians suggested more elaborate systems of faculties, by 1800 the idea of three faculties of mind was standard in both Europe and America. Despite any disagreement about the etiology of insanity, physicians believed that it arose from derangement of these basic faculties. Even those who posited more than three, such as Rush, believed that insanity was the derangement of mental faculties.[6]

## Psychiatry in Embryo

During the first three decades of the nineteenth century, a growing body of medical literature reflected the growth of thought about insanity on the Continent, in Great Britain, and in the United States. American and British physicians were particularly influenced by the work of the French clinicians. Attracting particular attention were the humanitarian and scientific efforts of Philippe Pinel, though significant numbers of American physicians did not

study in Paris until the 1820s and 1830s. The early American literature on insanity consisted largely of summaries of French and
British publications, but these writings reflected an awakened interest in a class of patients who needed medical attention. Both
Theodric Romeyn Beck and Isaac Ray, pioneer American physicians of the mind, cited Pinel and his French followers, J. E. D.
Esquirol, Étienne Georget, Jules Falret, the British James Cowles
Prichard, John Haslam, and John Conolly; and eclectically repeated the case histories found in them all. Americans, in addition,
used their own cases to illustrate and corroborate the observations
of the French and British writers, but the bulk of the cases they
recounted were still European.

Despite a common conceptual framework, clinicians disagreed
substantially about the clinical consequences of derangement of
the individual faculties and the relationship of one deranged faculty upon the others. Such lack of consensus among even the most
learned of observers led to difficulties in naming various disorders
as well as disagreements about whether these truly existed or were
a figment of theory. Clinicians agreed empirically, but their interpretations invited discussion, both among clinical observers and
particularly among the legal experts who more and more sought
their expertise.

### French Empirical Psychiatry

Pinel's work marked the application of clinical empiricism to
psychiatry. The publication of *Traité medicophilosophique sur l'alienation mentale ou la manie* in 1801 was the starting point of French,
German, and, to a great extent, British and American specialized
clinical psychiatry. Especially after the translation of this book
into English in 1806, its ideas were diffused widely in the United
States and Great Britain.

Pinel's methods of observation and study of the evolution of
patients' symptoms resulted in the discrimination of dangerousness as one critical feature of insanity among others. He believed
it was necessary to recognize potentially dangerous lunatics and

to have a method of preventing harm. He contended that the potential for dangerousness existed in only certain types of insanity.[7]

Pinel followed the faculty psychology of the day. He classified the various forms of mental derangement as defects of the intellect, the passions, and the will. He called derangement of the intellect "Melancholia." Among those patients were "deluded and dangerous beings who can commit most barbarous homicides in cold blood. Religious fanatics often fancy themselves inspired under divine requisition to perform some sacrificial act or acts of expiation."[8] In "mania without delirium," the lunatic exhibited no defect in the intellect, but was subject to fits of maniacal fury. One individual, the only son of a weak and indulgent mother, was perpetually embroiled in disputes and quarrels. Although in the management of his personal estate he was able to exercise sound judgment, he was eventually condemned to perpetual confinement at Bicêtre because he had become enraged with a woman who had used offensive language to him and "precipitated her into a well."[9]

Pinel warned that the most dangerous lunatics were those who were subject to sudden explosions of maniacal fury. He believed that they were the most difficult to manage because they suffered no intellectual derangement. Because they appeared to be sane, they were unpredictable and dangerous. During the French Revolution, brigands broke into the Bicêtre under the pretense of emancipating political prisoners. A maniac, bound in chains, convinced the mob of his sanity. The physician was compelled by circumstance to release him, though he warned the liberators of the man's disease. His fury aroused by the sight of so many armed men, the maniac grabbed the saber of one of the men and wounded several others.[10]

Pinel had observed that some lunatics could reason logically and yet be unable to control the passions or the will. Not all physicians would accept his authority on this point. The relationship of reason to responsibility would become a much debated issue in clinical and forensic psychiatry as the specialty evolved over the next few decades.

In accordance with his belief in the hazard of uncontrolled passions, Pinel did not hesitate to restrain dangerous individuals. If

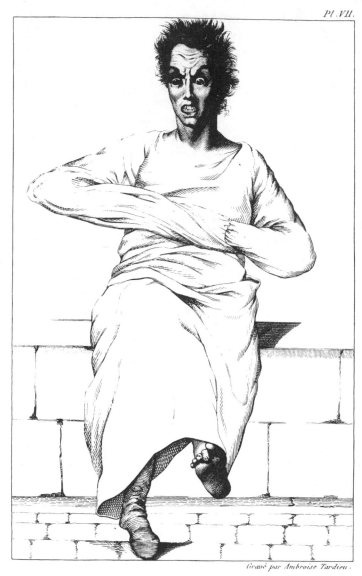

*Pl. VII.*

*Gravé par Ambroise Tardieu.*

Pinel warned that the most dangerous lunatics were those subject to sudden explosions of maniacal fury. J. E. D. Esquirol, *Des maladies mentales*, 1828. (Courtesy, Manuscripts and Rare Books Department, Swem Library, College of William and Mary) the physician could not control the maniacal fury or modify delusional ideation, then he should order mechanical restraint and seclusion in an isolation cell. Pinel did not advocate physical punishment in the management of dangerousness, but he did apply coercive methods to bring violent behavior under control.

### Americans After Pinel

Theodric Romeyn Beck's *Inaugural Dissertation on Insanity* of 1811 reflected the growing attention of American medical men to the care of the insane. The former relied upon Pinel's ideas about medical care and moral treatment. Beck had no training with the insane as a part of his medical education; he stated from the outset that the content of the dissertation was "information chiefly from books." Reflecting both French empiricism and the humanitarian reforms of the Quakers, he outlined the principal assumptions and practices of moral treatment, emphasizing the absolute authority of the physician and the capacity of lunatics to control their own behavior. He identified the unruly and dangerous: "If unruly, forbid them the company of others, use the straightcoat, confine them in a dark and quiet room, order a spare diet, and if danger is apprehended, apply metalic [*sic*] manacles to their hands and feet, as they are found not to injure by friction so much as linen or cotton.[11]

Beck believed that involuntary commitment was necessary for both the security of the public and for proper treatment. If an asylum were not available, then lunatics were to be confined in the home or some other safe place. Beck did not think that all lunatics were dangerous, but he believed they were "all more or less liable" to commit crimes for which they could not be held responsible.[12]

### Benjamin Rush

Dangerousness was not a conspicuous theme in Benjamin Rush's *Medical Inquiries and Observations upon the Diseases of the Mind* (1812). Of the several forms of mental derangement that he identified, none included dangerousness as a critical feature. Under the designation "Partial Intellectual Derangement," for example, he described various forms of the delusion, but he did not specify dangerousness in connection with any of them. Of "General Intellectual Derangement," namely mania, manicula, and manalgia, dangerousness was predicted only in the case of manalgia, in which the moral faculties became impaired and the patient became mischievous or vicious. In the first grade of intellectual derangement, mania, Rush continued, the madman "sometimes attempts to injure himself or others. Even inanimate objects . . . partake of his rage."[13]

Rush regarded murder and theft as symptoms or derangement of the will: "When the will becomes the involuntary vehicle of vicious actions, through the instrumentality of the passions, I have called it *Moral Derangement*." He believed that murder and theft, as well as lying and drinking, were symptoms of disease and that the former two should be "rescued" from the law by "the kind and lenient hand of medicine."[14]

## Rush's Classification

American writers on insanity were more attentive to the classification of the French than to Rush's, though his clinical empiricism was consistent with that of Pinel, Esquirol, and their Continental and British followers. The ideas of "partial" and "moral" insanity represented observations corroborated by other clinicians in works to follow, but the ideas themselves were a source of controversy well into the twentieth century. These new categories of insanity introduced new conceptualizations of dangerous lunacy.

That a person could behave normally and yet have thoughts and feelings that would overpower reason was a new idea and one not readily integrated into the Enlightenment way of thinking. Further, such lunatics were not readily diagnosed; physicians recognized the necessity of clinical training in mental diseases in order to identify and manage these individuals. A few British and Americans sought this training in France with Esquirol.

### Parkman Follows Pinel

George Parkman, the first American to study under Pinel and Esquirol in Paris, owned a private asylum in Massachusetts and became a strong advocate of lunacy reform and moral treatment. In 1817 his *Management of Lunatics, with Illustrations of Insanity* was published. It reflected Pinel's understanding of the dangerousness of lunatics and his management techniques. Parkman reported the tragedy of Captain James Purington, of Augusta, Maine, who in 1806 murdered his entire family because he believed that they would perish of starvation in the drought that year. Parkman used the case to illustrate the significance of delusions as a predictor of homicidal insanity. But, in the rest of the book as well as in his proposals for the establishment of his asylum, published in 1814, he followed Pinel faithfully.[15]

### Pinel's Influence on Early Jurisprudence of Insanity

Beck's second psychiatric book, *Elements of Medical Jurisprudence* (1823), was the first authoritative one on medical jurisprudence published in the United States. He again continued to reflect Pinel's influence as he had in 1811. In the chapter on "Mental Alienation," Beck attributed dangerousness to melancholy, as had Pinel, and gave the term a meaning like Pinel's:

It is while laboring under this that they become dangerous to themselves and to those around them. They will seize any weapon, and strike or injure others or themselves. Sometimes, consciousness of their situation is so far present as to allow them to warn individuals of their danger, or to entreat them to prevent their doing injury. An internal sensation is perceived—as a burning heat with pulsation within the skull—previous to this excitement."[16]

Beck did not differentiate between conscious and unconscious states. Later, he used the term "mania without delirium," within the context of discussing the difficulties of making a certain diagnosis of insanity in cases where the reason appeared to be unaffected. He stated, "But it is to be feared, that cases may sometimes occur, in which the dividing line between sanity and insanity may be overlapped, in the ardor to punish a foul homicide. The form of insanity which most commonly leads to the perpetration of this enormity, is one that assists in increasing the difficulty. It is that of melancholy, where the mind broods over a single idea, and that idea may be his own destruction or [that of] others."[17]

Beck's interest in lunacy was academic; he never directly cared for asylum patients. Nevertheless, *Elements of Medical Jurisprudence* went through successive editions. Beck became a member of the board of managers of the New York State Lunatic Asylum in 1842 and its president in 1854. Moreover, he edited the *American Journal of Insanity* for four years after the death of Amariah Brigham and gained recognition as an expert in the field.[18]

### Dangerousness in the Clinical Literature

Between 1825 and 1835, the French and English alienist physicians published a body of literature, mostly forensic, to which most of the ideas and controversies about dangerousness in American psychiatry could be traced for the rest of the century. In France, J. E. D. Esquirol and his student Étienne Georget published monographs on the medical jurisprudence of insanity. In 1828 Esquirol published *Des maladies mentales*. The principal British alienists, John Conolly and James Cowles Prichard, cited Esquirol and Georget extensively in treatises. Conolly and Prichard had read the works of the phrenologists Franz Joseph Gall and his follower Johann Christolph Spurzheim.[19]

### John Conolly and the Prediction of Dangerousness

In England, John Conolly was a major figure in the rise of psychiatry and an advocate of reform in the care of the insane. In 1830, before he had obtained any direct experience, his *An Inquiry concerning the Indications of Insanity with Suggestions for the Better Protection and Care of the Insane* was published. He had read Pinel, Esquirol, as well as Falret and drew his clinical examples largely from the French experience. He had gained substantial experience as a general practitioner and clinical instructor, which made him keenly

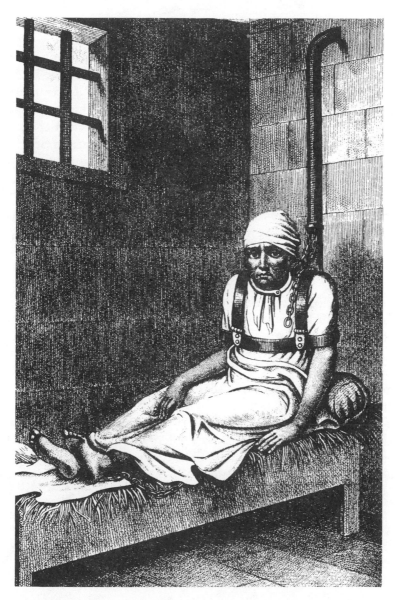

Early alienists did not hesitate to restrain lunatics whom they believed were dangerous. J. E. D. Esquirol, *Des maladies mentales*, 1828. (Courtesy, Manuscripts and Rare Books Department, Swem Library, College of William and Mary)

aware of the need for general physicians to be able to recognize and deal with cases of insanity.

Conolly believed in the organic nature of insanity and in individual faculties located in discrete anatomical sites. But he carried this theoretical explanation further to its dynamic implication: impairment of one or more faculties could induce a defect in the "comparing powers" of the mind. This particular conception was important to his understanding of delusion and, consequently, to his assessment of potential homicide. True, he said, various individual faculties of mind could become impaired, but such a condition would not necessarily constitute insanity. He asserted, "It must be remembered, that no propensity, however powerful, can produce madness, until it has either affected the sense, or the memory, or the imagination, or one or more of them; so as to disqualify the individual from exercising the powers of comparing."[20]

Conolly theorized further about the dynamics of delusions and homicide: "That which is false is believed, not because in these instances, that which is true is forgotten, for that which is true is believed also. . . . In this intellectual disorder, lunatics have committed atrocious crimes, feeling remorse even whilst committing them."[21] His belief that the faculties were located in various anatomical sites led Conolly to suggest that morbid excitation of the individual sites could give rise to morbid symptoms without total insanity. Such an irritation had led, he said, to the sudden desire to murder and destroy. He further noted that "men and women have cruely [sic] murdered their relatives, or even their own children, apparently impelled to such frightful crimes by a physical excitement, which was not extended to other propensities."[22] In addition to the direct irritation of nervous tissue in the brain, irritation from other parts of the body, particularly the gastrointestinal system, could, he believed, precipitate such a paroxysm.

### Conolly's Method of Assessing Dangerousness

Conolly specified that not all lunatics were dangerous. He emphasized the importance of direct and immediate examination, even though the physician may feel deterred by the "uncertain and dangerous movements of the lunatic."[23] Conolly said that the first part of the question was strictly a medical one, that of assessing the intellectual faculties, appearance, dress, words, actions, and the "known physical accompaniments of madness." But the second question was a medico-legal one, and it concerned the matter of interfering with the patient's civil rights. That the patient was delusional and hallucinating was diagnostic only of insanity; Conolly asserted that the content of the delusion had to be elicited in order for the physician to make the medico-legal judgment.

Conolly identified the delusional content that was to be considered a predictor of dangerousness. In addition to the well-defined delusion of persecution, he included patients who believed they were immortal or indestructible; those who would kill their children to save them from the wickedness of the world; and those who would murder in order to have themselves executed. In this context, Conolly discussed the issue of feigning; he concluded that even in cases of apparently insane murder, motiveless and gruesome, the perpetrator may not necessarily be insane.

### Restraint of Dangerous Lunatics

Conolly differentiated between "watching and superintendence" and restraint. The first of these could inform the doctor if and when the second was necessary. But, once the patient had revealed thoughts that threatened others or himself with bodily danger, then restraint was indicated. Conolly asserted:

The looks, or the language, or some outrage already committed, commonly reveal this character of the malady in cases in which it prevails; and once it is revealed, everything that security demands must be resorted to, and preserved in until the danger is past. To say when the danger *is*, is one of the most difficult things among the responsibilities of practicing among the insane.[24]

In order to avoid accidents, however, Conolly advised against reluctance to confine doubtful cases or failure to take action. He advised that precautions should be taken until the intellectual content of the disturbance was assessed.

Conolly regarded idiots capable of violence because they were unable to control their behavior. He believed that the will remained, but that it was under the control of depraved sensations and emotions, "from passions inordinate and unrestrained." He believed that idiots should be under perpetual restraint "because their liberty would be incompatible with the security of other persons."[25]

### Homicidal Insanity as a Rare Phenomenon

Conolly's treatment of dangerousness was scattered throughout his theoretical discussion of the nature of insanity and his practical advice concerning the duties of the physician in such cases. He did not believe that all lunatics were dangerous. He identified what he believed were the predictors of such a state. He maintained that treatment that involved restraint, however, was medico-legal in scope and went beyond the boundaries of strictly medical practice.

In 1856 Conolly wrote *The Treatment of the Insane without Mechanical Restraints*, after he had gained substantial experience at Hanwell Asylum, a 1,000-bed institution. He persisted in his original ideas about dangerousness. He did not, for example, permit delusional patients to walk unattended in the airing courts, for they could mistake others as "objects of his suspicion and dislike." His experience at the asylum confirmed his belief that "violent attacks, serious accidents, even homicides, have been the consequence of such delusions."[26]

### James Cowles Prichard and Moral Insanity

In addition to Conolly, American alienists read James Cowles Prichard, whose principal book on insanity was published in 1835. He had already published a volume on the diseases of the nervous system in 1822, a result of his work in general medicine at St. Peter's Hospital. He exerted a major influence upon the medical jurisprudence of insanity and was one of the first Commissioners in Lunacy in Great Britain.[27] His special contribution was the concept of "moral insanity."

Prichard claimed to have identified moral insanity as a distinct illness. Esquirol disagreed with him. In his 1838 work, Esquirol said, "Doct. Prichard has not, perhaps sufficiently distinguished *moral insanity* from another variety, which is also exempt from disorder of the understanding, and which Pinel denominates mania without delirium."[28] However, Prichard believed that Pinel's concept, also called "homicidal monomania" by Georget and Esquirol, was only one type of moral insanity. The critical feature of this phenomenon, according to Prichard, was that the intellect could remain intact. He defined this type of moral insanity as "a contest in the mind of the individual between the instinctive desire which constitutes the whole manifestation of the disease, and the judgement of the understanding still unaffected and struggling against it."[29] As historian of science Roger Smith has explained it, Pinel and Esquirol had already created a "medical orthodoxy" that insane violence could be accompanied by rational and moral judgement.[30] Prichard explained the phenomenon in terms of a lesion of the moral propensity; in moral insanity, the feelings were not controlled by the intellect: "The sudden anger of a person labouring under moral insanity, and subject to paroxysms of rage . . . [was] an immediate impulse arising spontaneously on the mind, which was diseased only in its moral constitution."[31]

### Esquirol's Three Types of Homicidal Insanity

The cases that Prichard used to illustrate his idea of moral insanity were those, in fact, from Pinel, Esquirol, Georget, C. C. H. Marc, and the English courts. But Esquirol had identified three subtypes of homicidal monomania: (1) intellectual monomania, in which the intellectual disorder was confined to a single or limited number of ideas (this type of disorder was later called paranoia); (2) affective monomania (reasoning mania), in which lunatics made use of their reason while the affections and dispositions were perverted (later psychopathic personality); and (3) instinctive monomania, where a lesion of the will existed and the reason and emotions were powerless to control the behavior (later irresistible impulse). Prichard, at first, did not differentiate among Esquirol's three ways in which the intellect could remain intact.[32]

Prichard subsequently modified his thinking about the role of the intellect in moral insanity. In his second work, published in 1842, he clarified this point. Noting Esquirol's objections to his original conception, he defined moral insanity as a "disorder which affects only the feelings and affections." He defined monomania as "intellectual aberration or delusion . . . superadded to the phenomenon or moral insanity." Finally, he identified the insane impulse as a separate entity.[33] His conceptions covered the faculties of intellect, emotion, and volition.

By the mid-1830s, the organizing principle of faculty psychology dominated psychiatric thought and explained clinical observations. Yet, clinicians noted other phenomena that did not fit neatly into their conceptual framework. The celebrated case of Henriette Cornier is an example of a type of insanity that had not been accounted for in the predominant classification and confounded the alienists as well as the French medico-legal experts who were involved in the case.

Henriette Cornier, a domestic servant, with planning and without remorse, killed a child of nineteen months. Henriette persuaded the mother, a friend of her employer, to allow her to take the child out for a walk. But, instead, she took the little girl to the home of her employer, beheaded her, and threw the head into the street when the mother came to pick up the child. Henriette demonstrated no emotion or grief, and "to all that was said she replied, with indifference, "J'ai voulu le tuer!"

The case was widely publicized in France. Esquirol was among those alienists who repeatedly examined Cornier, both before the trial and after she was committed to the Sâlpetrière for observation. She had committed the murder with clear intellect and emotional indifference, but had been impelled by a powerful impulse. "J'ai eu une idée," she replied when pressed further by her examiners. Esquirol testified that she suffered from instinctive monomania. Despite his reputation, the jury's verdict was that Cornier had committed the homicide voluntarily, but without premeditation. She was condemned to perpetual imprisonment with forced labor.[34]

Not all of the alienists who testified in the case believed, as Esquirol did, that such a phenomenon as instinctive monomania existed. On the other hand, few felt that Cornier was sane, though no consensus could be reached about the true nature of the insanity. But the case demonstrated that not all insanity was characterized by an impairment of the intellect.

### Isaac Ray and American Forensic Psychiatry

The major work of Isaac Ray, an American who became a major figure in world forensic psychiatry, was published before the debate between Prichard and Esquirol. Like Esquirol, Ray had some difficulty with Prichard's original conception of moral insanity. For the most part, Ray's book was informed by Esquirol's thought, but also cited Georget, John Haslam, Conolly, and Prichard. Ray criticized from the outset the laws of both the United States and Great Britain as "loose, vacillating, and greatly behind the present state of knowledge of that disease insanity." He rejected the criterion of the delusion as the legal test for insanity. He asserted, "Insanity is a disease, and as is the case with all other diseases, the fact of existence is never established by a single diagnostic symptom, but by the whole body of symptoms, no particular one of which is present in every case."[35]

Ray accepted the existence of subtle and varying grades of insanity based upon his belief in the topology of discrete faculties and propensities in cerebral tissue. He contended that the cerebral tissues could become diseased, could be congenitally absent, or could be inadequately developed. Because he believed that insanity was both a disease of specific anatomical sites and a disease of varying intensities, he attributed dangerousness to a broad range of mental disorders.

### Ray and the Moral Faculty

Ray's conceptual framework was the same as Prichard's. The former believed that the clinical features of insanity were the result of either attenuated or irritated intellectual faculties. He maintained that any condition that affected the function of the moral faculty made the patient dangerous. The idiot and the imbecile, for example, were especially dangerous if the moral faculty was congenitally absent, weak, or perverted. Ray agreed with Prichard on the idea of moral insanity: perversions of the moral faculty could occur in the presence of adequate intelligence. If, by some pathological process in the brain, the moral faculty became impaired, Ray used the term "moral mania."[36]

In all these instances, Ray believed that predictable danger existed. He noted, "By imbecility is ordinarily understood a deficiency of the intellect; but it has been seen . . . that its signification is here extended to include that class of subjects in whom mental defect consists in a great deficiency, if not utter destitution of the higher *moral* faculties."[37]

Ray reported the case of John Schmidt as an example. At the age of seventeen, the boy was tried and condemned to death at Metz for parricide. He had a childhood history of cruel mischief-making and practical jokes that often resulted in injury or near-death. In one of these incidents, he nearly drowned his cousin. He had also tried to murder his sister-in-law, and he finally did kill his parents. He confessed to his counsel that "whenever he saw a cutting instrument such as a hatchet, a knife etc., he felt the strongest desire to seize it, and wound the first person that came his way." Ray interpreted the case as follows: "His inclination to kill on seeing a cutting instrument, shows some morbid action in the brain not uncommon in imbecility, which is also indicated by the paroxysm of fury in which he felt himself urged on to indiscriminate slaughter. . . . His extraordinary proneness to mischief and cruelty, and at the early age at which it began to appear, point distinctly to an original defect of constitution."[38]

Ray cited a similar illustration from Georget, one Pierre Joseph Delephine, age sixteen, who received a death sentence, later commuted to life imprisonment, for eight different incendiary acts. Ray concluded that the only safe management course for the moral imbecile was perpetual confinement, "which at once secures society from their future aggressions, and is most conducive to their mental and bodily welfare."[39]

Ray believed that the brain could, like any other organ of the body, undergo pathological changes. He asserted, *"Insanity observes the same pathological laws as other diseases."*[40] He suggested that the whole moral nature could be thrown into chaotic confusion, or only one or two of the moral powers affected, depending upon the extent of the physical irritation. Ray differentiated between Pinel's *manie sans délire* and Prichard's moral insanity on account of his belief that discrete areas of pathology in the brain tissue caused different forms of mental disease because individual faculties were affected. Esquirol wrote of "lesions" of intelligence, affections, or will, but he did not postulate precise anatomical sites for such faculties. Ray, by contrast, believed in general and partial involvement in the concrete sense.[41]

### Multiple Moral Faculties

In Ray's conceptual framework, the degree of dangerousness in the morally insane lunatic depended upon which of the moral faculties was involved in the pathology. He contended, "Exaltation of the vital forces" in any part of the brain led to "increased activity and energy in the manifestations of the faculty connected with it." He believed impulses were morbid symptoms caused by pathology of these discrete sites. Depending upon the propensity involved, the impulse could be benign, such as the "inordinate propensity to lying," or dangerous, such as the "homicidal impulse." In this way, he accounted for the lunatic who was compelled to kill someone by an imperative idea, such as Henriette Cornier. Ray also believed that the same pathology could cause homicidal monomania, that is, premeditated killing as a result of delusions.[42]

Ray's thinking is particularly significant because it was a practical synthesis of the predominant ideas in France and England about the clinical empiricist descriptions of insanity and the need for humanitarian reforms based upon this progress, especially in recognizing criminal insanity in its various forms. Ray's book also reflects the inconsistencies of classification and the failure among alienists to reach consensus about issues basic to the medico-legal relationship. This book marked Ray as knowledgeable in matters of lunacy (though he wrote nothing about its medical treatment), and he was offered the superintendency of the Maine Insane Asylum in 1841. Over the next forty years, as an asylum superintendent and reformer, he exercised substantial influence, but he did not change his essential ideas about dangerousness.[43]

Ray, whose influence in psychiatry persisted through the nineteenth century, maintained a series of beliefs that pertained to dangerousness in the following way: (1) He organized his observations around the conceptual framework of faculty psychology; (2) Like Esquirol and Prichard, he believed that the brain itself was diseased, but he further posited discrete anatomical sites, and the pathology of these cells accounted for the different forms and intensities of derangement; and (3) He claimed that dangerousness originated in the pathology of specific propensities that were anatomically discrete. His ideas, therefore, reflected English, French, and American experiences and belief, except for the anatomical loci, which had their origin at least in part in phrenology.

### Phrenology and Insane Homicide

The idea that the brain was a composition of discrete anatomical organs was basic to American and British psychiatry during the first four decades of the nineteenth century. Such thinking owed much, as has been suggested, to phrenology. Franz Joseph Gall, the founder of this discipline, was a German physician who was particularly influenced by the work of Giovanni Batista Morgagni, the Italian pathologist. The idea of organ pathology informed Gall's theory; Dain has noted that the modifications by Spurzheim made phrenology more acceptable to American alienists. Spurzheim's work appeared in two American editions, 1832 and 1836, which explicitly and directly affected American and British psychiatric thinking.[44]

Eric T. Carlson has noted that Americans who were particularly influenced by phrenology—Amariah Brigham, Isaac Ray, Charles H. Steadman—rejected the craniological aspects of phrenology and were skeptical about the organology. The idea that the con-

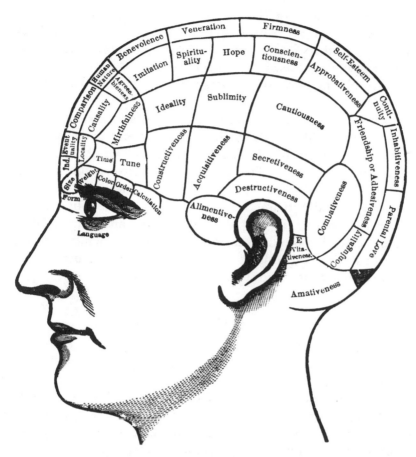

Names, Numbers and Location of the Mental Organs. Lydia F. Fowler, *Familiar Lessons on Phrenology*, 1848. (Courtesy, Swem Library, College of William and Mary)

dition of the brain could be improved by education was fundamental to the moral treatment most Americans advocated. But
they also felt that insanity was a disease of the brain as well as a
very complicated disease. This supported the need for medical in-
tervention in the preventive, therapeutic, and public aspects of insanity.[45]

Alienists consistently ignored the doctrinaire aspects of phrenology, but Spurzheim's clinical observations were consistent
with those of alienists who were gaining their initial experiences
in the care of the insane. The concept of discrete organs or faculties
of mind was consistent with the asylum clinical experience and
followed logically from Scottish common-sense philosophy.[46]
Esquirol, Conolly, and Ray did not mention anything about the
external cranial configuration in relation to the faculties, though
Esquirol measured crania of normal, insane, and mentally defective women in an isolated study.[47]

## Organ of Destructiveness

Spurzheim postulated a simple explanation for dangerousness. In
the 1822 American edition of his major work on phrenology, he
diagrammed the location of the various faculties and described the
discrete organs, one of which was the "Organ of Destructiveness."
He assigned the propensity to kill to this organ. He reasoned that
the inherent energy of this propensity determined whether car-
nivorous animals limited their killing to certain species for food
and whether they killed for the pleasure of it. In humans, he postulated, great sensitivity or gross indifference, even pleasure, were
created by the sufferings of other beings. A highly active Organ
of Destructiveness led people to enjoy public executions, the
slaughter of animals, and battles.

The inherent energy of the Organ of Destructiveness was independent of education and/or social breeding. Spurzheim cited
many cases from all levels of society to support his idea that "this
terrible propensity is sometimes quite independent of education,
of example, or of habit, and that it depends on innate constitution
alone. Many crimes are so detestable, and are accompanied with

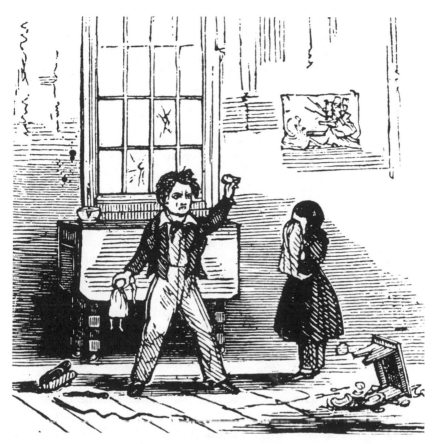

The Faculty of Destructiveness. Gall named this propensity the "Organ of Murder" because he had found it to be of large size in the skulls of two murderers. Spurzheim believed that Destructiveness was essential to human existence. Lydia F. Fowler, *Familiar Lessons on Phrenology*, 1848. (Courtesy, Swem Library, College of William and Mary)

such repugnant and horrible circumstances, that it would be impossible to explain them in any other way." Spurzheim even cited cases of cannibalism in this context and claimed that this propensity was often highly active in idiots.[48]

## Organ of Murder

Gall had named the Organ of Destructiveness the "Organ of Murder" because he had found its location to be predominant in the skulls of two murderers. Spurzheim disagreed with Gall on the naming of the organ. Spurzheim believed that the Organ of Destructiveness was essential to human existence; for the continuation of humanity, it was necessary to destroy what was useless or hurtful, and it was sometimes necessary and lawful for individuals to destroy other humans to preserve themselves. The basic nature and purpose of the Organ of Destructiveness was self-preservation.[49]

The existence of homicidal insanity of any clinical type was the result of derangement of this single propensity. Spurzheim described various cases of lunatics who were seized by the homicidal impulse. Overactivity of the propensity could be accompanied by delusions; in this way, Spurzheim accounted for homicidal monomania. He cited cases in this context from Pinel in which lunatics had killed under the influence of delusions and command hallucinations. The morbid impulse and "periodic fits of fury" that led to homicide were also caused, according to Spurzheim, by overactivity of this propensity. The phrenologists' suggestion that all homicidal insanity was reducible to the derangement of a localized anatomical site located "immediately above the ear" was too simplistic in view of the clinical observations already accumulated by 1830. But the idea of a site that could undergo pathological changes was, of course, consistent with current medical thinking.

The Organ of Destructiveness was absent from Spurzheim's first American edition of *Observations on the Deranged Manifestations of the Mind, or Insanity*, published in 1833. In the context of the discussion of derangement of the feelings, he said, "Murderous impulse, however unaccountable it may appear to others, is not always obedient to will." He cited Pinel's case of Thomas Callaby, who in 1805 murdered his grandchild and wounded his wife under the influence of the homicidal impulse.[50] Pinel had called it a derangement of the will.

In the context of derangement of the intellectual faculties, Spurzheim identified the existence of delusional states that could propel the patient to homicide, but he did not cite any clinical cases to illustrate the assertion. The sole example he used was that of the hypothetical "maniac [who] took for a legion of devils every assemblage of people he saw."[51] Like other writers of the day, Spurzheim accounted for delusions in terms of either excitement or of suppression of the intellectual faculty.

Amariah Brigham, whose interest in insanity led him eventually to an asylum superintendency, edited Spurzheim's 1833 edition and added his own appendix. Brigham did not necessarily ascribe dangerousness to any specific locus. He said in the appendix under the heading "Monomania" that the system of phrenology explained cases of partial insanity better than any other. Brigham did not take note here of Spurzheim's inconsistency. In his own treatment of the subject of suicide, Brigham wrote of self-destruction and suicide pacts of two people. Yet, he made no reference at all to homicidal insanity in connection with suicide and no mention of the organs of Cautiousness and Destructiveness, which, according to Spurzheim, were deranged in such a form of insanity. Brigham, furthermore, discussed the moral, or circumstantial, causes of suicide.[52]

Brigham also edited the American edition of Andrew Combe's *Observations on Mental Derangement: Being an Application of the Principles of Phrenology to the Elucidation of the Causes, Symptoms, Nature, and Treatment of Insanity* (1834). Combe and his brother, George, a barrister, were both passionate followers of Spurzheim and proselytizers of phrenology, and yet Andrew said, "Whether we adopt an Organ of Destructiveness in the brain or not, it is to be assumed that the propensity to kill . . . arose from a morbid excitation of a certain part of the brain."[53]

Combe listed the "fundamental principles of the new physiology of the brain," which were Spurzheim's organology and craniology, but in an introductory essay he recognized that the doctrinal facets of phrenology were accepted by medical men with reservations or not at all. In fact, Combe himself was at first skeptical of phrenology, but based his acceptance upon accumulated clinical evidence. He had studied with Esquirol in Paris and relied upon Esquirol's clinical data. But, unlike Esquirol, Combe frequently went beyond the data to conclusions impossible to confirm or deny given the status of brain research in the 1830s. The theoretical attraction of phrenology for Combe, Brigham, and other thinkers was that it posited a somatic explanation for mental phenomena.[54]

### Insanity and Medical Science

As the foregoing survey of leading thinkers shows, during the first forty years of the nineteenth century in the United States physicians claimed that the study of insanity was a part of medical science. In Europe, Great Britain, and the United States, reformers established benevolent institutions for the care of the insane, and clinical experience began to accumulate. Much of the clinical data upon which early American and British theoretical writing was founded came from the French. These observations, however, were corroborated by Parkman, Beck, and Ray in the United States as well as Conolly and Prichard in Great Britain. Gall and Spurzheim also found evidence among these data to support the theory of phrenology.

Because of their clinical experience, physicians also began to classify insanity into subtypes and various diseases. By the 1830s the idea that the brain could be partially affected was widely accepted, thus calling for refined diagnostic techniques and individual prescriptions. Even before the development of asylum practice, physicians took seriously their power to deprive their fellow citizens of liberty and called for careful assessment of the individual lunatic. In theory, at least, they believed that only the dangerously insane should be locked up, either by mechanical devices or in seclusion cells. Alienists perceived a clear difference in theory and practice between restraint in the application of the moral treatment and restraint applied in the service of protecting others from the dangerous lunatic. In theory, also, only a small proportion of the insane were homicidal.

Between 1800 and 1840, the idea of individual faculties of mind and phrenological ideas about discrete mental organs supported the conceptual framework synthesized by the observations of all these psychiatric writers. Although classification was uncertain as well as variable and some celebrated cases of insane homicide did not fall neatly into the diagnostic framework, the French clinical empiricists established a medical orthodoxy in which treatment of the varying and subtle forms of insanity was clearly the responsibility of medical professionals.

# The Development of a Medical Jurisprudence of Insanity   **3**

Concurrent with the growth of psychiatry as a medical specialty in the mid-nineteenth century, medico-legal experts began to address the issue of insane homicide within the context of involuntary commitment, criminal proceedings, and release from the asylum. At no time during this early asylum period did physicians believe that all mentally ill people were dangerous. The readiness to commit persons diagnosed as insane was not based upon the prediction of dangerousness, but upon the belief that they were in need of protection and refuge.

Between 1840 and 1869, the asylum approach to psychiatry was established and came to a brief fruition; then flaws became apparent. This approach disappointed proponents because it was founded upon the assumption that the insane could be cured by their prompt dispatch to the controlled environment of the asylum. It is true that they often improved substantially with classic moral management. But the founders of the specialty did not have the opportunity to test the hypothesis or to improve the method. Early in the asylum period, the ideal of a controlled environment became more and more difficult to achieve. Buildings crumbled, destructive lunatics destroyed the decor, and single rooms became dormitories as the need for room outstripped the capacity of the institution to maintain the tasteful environment that was essential for providing the moral treatment.[1]

But, even after medical superintendents accepted the reality that insanity was not cured merely by the asylum environment, these institutions continued to be built, expanded, and funded because they met social needs, not the least of which was to isolate the insane, whom people believed could be dangerous. Between 1860 and 1870, the practice of psychiatry was plagued not only by internal theoretical disagreements, but also by challenges from outside the profession to the authority of the asylum superintendent to commit and detain people. After 1870 the new medical specialty of neurology challenged the basic tenets of the asylum superintendents.[2]

The superintendents unhesitatingly identified the homicidal insane in their own institutions and exercised their prerogative to control them with mechanical restraints. But the authors of the annual reports of the early asylums devoted more attention to the number of suicidal patients in need of the watchful attention of the attendants than to the presence of homicidal lunatics. Although some of the patients were certainly dangerous, to have called attention to their presence would have militated against the therapeutic image of the asylum.[3] Later in the century, when asylums became grossly overcrowded, the presence of the homicidal insane would give rise to discussion and rhetoric about the "virtuous" and the "wicked" insane, along with a cry for separate establishments. The belief that the homicidal insane were essentially depraved and therefore deserving of some punishment still informed psychiatric thinking in some instances.

## The Alienist as Medico-Legal Expert

By 1840 physicians, and the public as well, associated insane homicide with distinct mental phenomena. In the spirit of the Enlightenment, more and more the medical superintendents were called upon by the courts to make discriminatory judgments about whether a murderer was a homicidal lunatic or merely a criminal.

Some superintendents, and later neurologists, particularly those who were guided by a religious devotion to the primacy of reason, ignored the empirical data and applied their own standards to the diagnostic process. Differences of theoretical opinion surfaced in medico-legal cases in which alienists publicly disagreed.[4]

Experts in the jurisprudence of insanity generally agreed about the concepts of partial insanity (homicidal monomania, homicidal impulse, moral insanity) postulated by Esquirol and Prichard, though speculation prevailed about whether or not the intellect could remain intact in any insanity. When Forbes Winslow, the British alienist, wrote *The Plea of Insanity in Criminal Cases* (1843), he recognized the existence of partial insanity and monomania (that is, delusions without other signs, such as disorientation and hallucinations), but he did not equate the two mental conditions. He was also adamant in his rejection of the existence of delusion as a test for insanity; in fact, he believed that no single test was available and that the lunatic's mental state could be assessed only within the context of its own history. Winslow disagreed with Prichard that the dangerous lunatic acts without motive: "Are not the insane often impelled to the commission of acts of violence and murder *by the same motives, feelings, and passions, that influence and regulate the conduct of sound, healthy, and rational minds.*"[5]

Winslow's thesis was that no legal test for insanity existed. The diagnosis of homicidal insanity was a matter of cautious assessment of thought content. Winslow contended that the laws of both Great Britain and the United States were inadequate for the various instances in which insane homicide could occur. Fully agreeing with Prichard on the issue of moral insanity, he remarked "The gallows ends the career of many a moral maniac."[6]

The search for a certain test for insanity was an important issue for the courts. Alienists devised individual techniques for assessing mental status. In differentiating between the homicidal insane and the mere criminal, some alienists made qualitative judgments about impairment of individual faculties; others, like Winslow, for example, conceived of insanity quantitatively, in terms of degree rather than kind. For most alienists, the term partial insanity could mean either intermittent insanity or insanity limited to certain mental faculties. Undoubtedly, these two methods of conceptualizing insanity complicated the process of arriving at a unitary concept of dangerousness either theoretically or in a court of law. Like Winslow, the British medical jurist Alfred S. Taylor treated partial insanity quantitatively. He believed that it was unlikely that moral insanity ever existed without some degree of disorder of the intellectual faculty. "It is not sufficient to seek merely for evidence of delusion," he said, "it is our business to consider how far that may endanger the well-being of himself and his friends."[7] Taylor demanded a definable change in character or overt threats.

Beck, now editor of the *American Journal of Insanity* after Brigham's death, reviewed Taylor's book in the July 1845, issue. Of Taylor's position on involuntary restraint and the quantitative assessment of delusions, Beck commented:

The greatest abuses of the restraint system are said to have occurred in respect to monomania, in which individuals have been forcibly imprisoned because they entertained some absurd delusions. . . . But the main and important point of interest [in Taylor's treatment of involuntary commitment] is not even hinted at. It is, whether some mode cannot be devised of preventing these awfully numerous cases of murder and suicide which are now a days perpetrated by monomaniacs, or in other words, by such as labor under *dangerous delusions*! . . . better that some hypochondriacs be temporarily secluded, than that a troop of homicidal and suicidal monomaniacs be allowed from day to day to work themselves up to the commitment of these enormities.[8]

Taylor maintained that past homicidal behavior was the most reliable predictor of dangerousness. Beck agreed: "One who has been guilty of a heinous crime like murder, should never, on any pretense, be discharged. There are often long lucid intervals in homicidal mania; and it is impossible to be certain that the disease is entirely removed."[9] Alienists had noted that, in some cases, long periods of perfect sanity were interposed between periods of madness. Although the law, according to Taylor, would hold lunatics responsible for crimes committed during lucid intervals, the prevailing medical opinion was that they were always subject to recurring "cerebral irritations." Taylor believed that the homicidal lunatic should always be considered dangerous.


## Judicial Removal of Dangerous Lunatics from Asylums

Alienists, medico-jurisprudents, and, incidentally, lawyers generally agreed upon the nature of homicidal insanity and the fact that homicidal lunatics should be incarcerated indefinitely. Although alienists were given the authority to restrain all the insane, in some jurisdictions the town magistrates retained the authority to release them from asylums for the purposes of economy. In 1848 Brigham reported three cases of unrestrained lunatics who committed homicides.[10]

The responsibility for retaining the dangerous lunatic in the asylum was squarely the medical superintendent's unless he was overpowered by the judicial system. Alienists were reluctant to pronounce any lunatic cured, least of all a homicidal one, in the face of the consequences that had ensued in a small number of cases. This dilemma contributed to the vast overcrowding of the asylums, beginning as early as the 1850s in some states. The problem of releasing recovering lunatics, whether homicidal or virtuous, would burgeon into open controversy in the Association during the 1870s.[11]

Between 1850 and 1890, however, the turmoil of criticism of the whole asylum system resulted in some restrictions being placed upon the alienists concerning involuntary commitments. Although they were authorized to commit all the insane on the principle of what Ray called "the great law of Humanity," in a few widely publicized instances patients sued them for false commitment. Personal accounts of unwarranted involuntary commitment inflamed the public's belief that alienists could exercise their power to commit perfectly sane persons to insane asylums through conspiracy.[12]

From an early date, doctors feared legal action for false commitment, a pressure counter to the apprehension involved with being held responsible for the actions of released patients. In 1863, for example, the editor of the *American Journal of Insanity* reported a case that reflected the predicament:

The prisoner was a married woman, twenty-one years of age, and four months advanced in pregnancy. She had been twice *enceinte* before, and during those periods had suffered from great despondency, and had always exhibited a peculiar horror of knives and razors. She murdered her child by cutting its throat, and then attempted her own life, first by wounding her throat, and then by throwing herself out of window [*sic*]. She also took laudanum, which was detected in some fluid she vomited. This at least appears to have been an instance where the catastrophe might have been foreseen and prevented. Yet, probably, any physician, who in her previous pregnancies had recommended restraint [,] would have had some difficulty in proving to a jury its necessity, if proceedings had been taken against him for wrongly signing the certificate of lunacy.[13]

Ray was particularly concerned about protecting alienists from legal action. By 1850 he had prepared for the Association a comprehensive law project covering every aspect of their legal relations with the insane. The project called for uniformity of statutes from state to state, based upon a psychiatric theory that itself was not uniform. Therefore, the consistency that Ray envisioned was never achieved. By the late 1880s, however, the legal principles underlying his thought were sufficiently established that both the rights of patients and the protection of alienists became part of the statutes of most states. But in the interim doctors were continually attacked by public opinion, both for instances of false commitment and the release of dangerous lunatics.[14]

## The Rise of Moral Somaticism

Up until the 1850s, American and British alienists did not perceive any methodological differences between clinical and moral judgments. Dain noted that American practitioners were never committed to Continental efforts to remove religious belief from the study of man. Therefore, in the United States, ideas about essential morality continued to exert a significant impact upon medico-legal decision-making.[15] Moral somaticism was the idea that only physical disease conferred the sick role upon lunatics, thereby absolving them of any moral responsibility for insane behavior.

This notion surfaced prominently in the mid-1850s. In 1855 John Purdue Gray assumed the editorship of the *American Journal of Insanity* and began a period of significant departure from the influence of the French clinical empiricists. He rejected the existence of separate faculties of mind on religious and philosophical grounds. He thereby rejected Esquirol's concept of monomania and Prichard's moral insanity, along with the idea that a person could be seized with transitory or impulsive states in the absence of physical disease. The mind, or soul, was a unitary entity.

Gray disagreed with Ray and others who believed that some subtle forms of insanity required prolonged assessment. For Gray, people were insane if they manifested a well-defined psychosis or suffered from physical illness that deranged their brains.[16] In the 1868 case of Mrs. Elizabeth Heggie, who was executed for poisoning both her daughters, he found her to be "cross, irritable, ugly and repulsive," but not delusional. Alienists George Cook and D. Tilden Brown testified that she was a monomaniac whose sole delusion was that her daughters were plotting to displace her in the family. Gray testified that he had never seen a case of monomania. Not only was there conflicting testimony among the alienists, but also between them and other nonexpert medical witnesses, unfortunately for Mrs. Heggie.[17]

Gray, however, recognized that the disposition to violence was a common characteristic of mental disease. In a paper read before the Association in May 1857, he analyzed fifty-two cases of homicide and attempted homicide as well as cases admitted to Utica Asylum, where he was medical superintendent, on the basis of predicted dangerousness. He rejected the idea of homicidal monomania or homicidal impulse:

That in insanity there is developed a disposition to extreme violence of murder, and that disposition is, at time, irresistible, no one familiar with the insane will for a moment pretend to doubt; . . . the homicidal act, in irresponsible persons, generally, if not always, has for its origin and development such disturbance of feelings as usually influence the sane to other carefully planned or sudden acts of violence; and that a full and reliable history or sudden or more or less persistent homicidal propensity will reveal the fact, that *in all instances*, anterior to any such impulse, there existed for a time physical *disease*. . . . The existence of the third class, in which the impulse is sudden and unreflected on, admits of grave doubt.[18]

If violence in mental illness were to take place, Gray asserted, it was the result of a disease that had a history. He stated that the idea of affective monomania was "one of those unhappy terms in medicine which, while it aims to express the character of the peculiar cases intended to be included under it, it is rather the expression of a theory never yet fully established." He argued further that homicidal monomania was a part of the whole theory of moral insanity that was being questioned and rejected by Winslow, Bucknill, and others. "That such a form of insanity has been enunciated by Esquirol, or by other acknowledged authorities in the profession," he said, "is not in itself an evidence of its real existence." For Gray, moral insanity and homicidal monomania were mere excuses for crime.[19]

As a representative of the moral somaticist standpoint, Gray was not denying the existence of insanity in, for example, Henriette Cornier. She appeared to the alienists and to the courts to have retained the full use of her reason. But evidence of insanity, Gray maintained, was to be found in the existence of well-defined physical disease or in a change in the character of the emotional status of the lunatic prior to the homicide, a clearly defined finding in the case of Cornier.

The development of moral somaticism was greatly accelerated in 1856 with the publication of British alienists John Charles Bucknill and Daniel Hack Tuke's *A Manual of Psychological Medicine*, a comprehensive textbook of psychiatry that would pass through four editions between 1858 and 1879. The two men became the most cited authorities on clinical psychiatry during the next three decades.[20]

Gray had asserted that Bucknill had questioned the concept of moral insanity. Neither Bucknill nor Tuke denied the existence of moral insanity or of impulsive states. Their treatment of these issues throughout this textbook reflected the somaticist view, that diseases demonstrated an etiology, an onset, and an identifiable course that deviated from the patient's normal state. Bucknill asserted that "perhaps the only diagnostic symptom between mere vicious propensities and moral insanity, is the mode of causation."[21]

Moral somaticism was not incompatible with the idea of partial insanity. Tuke's classification of mental diseases reflected the traditional faculty psychology. Although he did not use the term "monomania" in the scheme, Esquirol's three types of monomania were implicit. Homicidal insanity could arise from derangement of any of the faculties. But Tuke maintained, "The existence of *Homicidal Insanity* ought never to be admitted without the proof of other symptoms of mental disease than the perverted instinct itself, or at least without the existence of well-recognized or efficient causes of mental disease, and an obvious change in the temper and disposition consequent thereupon."[22]

Bucknill and Tuke articulated the application of physical diagnosis to mental disease. If physical signs and symptoms could be elicited by the physician or the onset and course of the disease could be traced, then he gave moral absolution to the lunatic. This idea would play an important role in the prediction of dangerousness and the disposition of homicidal lunatics throughout the nineteenth and into the twentieth century.

# 4

## From Static Brain to Dynamic Neurophysiology 1840–1870

In 1840 the idea that insanity was disease of the brain was the starting point of all psychiatric theory and practice. Yet, the ultimate nature of the brain was subject to intense controversy and philosophical interpretation. Some physicians conceived of it as an aggregate of parts that could become individually or collectively deranged. Others imagined it to be a unitary organ that was never subject to partial pathologies. All agreed, however, that it was subject to irritation from the visceral organs and from moral causes, namely "bad living" and life's misfortunes.

Over the next thirty years, the idea that the brain was a static organ that was acted upon from without would change to the conception of the brain as a physiological dynamism. The new alienists would therefore reason that psychiatric patients were unpredictable and more universally dangerous than earlier physicians had believed.

### Intellectual Insanity: Homicidal Mania and Delusional Insanity

Alienists on both sides of the ocean disagreed about the fundamental issue of the power of the intellect to control behavior. For many years into the nineteenth century, the delusion had been the single diagnostic criterion of insanity because alienists and lawyers agreed that insanity was by definition derangement of the intellect. By the 1840s such a single criterion had been successfully challenged in theory and in practice, but derangement of the intellectual faculty, evidenced by false ideas, continued to serve as an unamibiguous symptom of insanity. Some alienists believed that any delusion made the patient dangerous, but for the most part, early clinicians had established the standard that it was the content of the delusion rather than the mere fact of its existence that made the patient dangerous.

The presence of hallucinations and illusions, though separate phenomena, were generally taken to be closely associated with the existence of delusion. In this context, therefore, homicidal mania or delusional insanity often meant that the patient exhibited delusions, hallucinations, and illusions. Delusional insanity therefore meant that the patient's intellectual faculty was impaired in the broadest sense.

### The Primacy of Reason

In 1844 Brigham interrogated more than twenty criminal lunatics on the subject of "right and wrong" and learned that they showed no defect of reason. He therefore argued that the homicidal impulse was a partial insanity:

Their opinions on the subject were correct [that it was wrong to steal and that murder was the greatest crime]; but still, the same individuals may be wholly unable to resist their diseased impulses, and therefore commit crimes they know to be wrong. Other deranged persons commit crimes from delusions, in obedience to supposed commands from others, or from on high; and although they know the act in itself is wrong, they dare not, and cannot disobey the command.[1]

Only the most naive clinicians could ignore cases of homicidal insanity characterized by remorselessness and impulsivity. Those who recognized the existence of such cases but who rejected the concept of partial insanity maintained that intellectual involvement was always present but overlooked. On the issue of behavioral control, Gray said that even in intellectual involvement the insane rarely lost their self-control, a fact that constituted the basis for moral treatment. He believed that this fact accounted for the observation that they could conceal their delusions.[2]

Moral somaticists who rejected separating the faculties of mind nevertheless recognized that one class of symptoms could predominate in insanity. But it followed, they reasoned, that all cases progressed eventually to dementia. They did not believe that the disease could remain stationary for long. At the 1863 meeting of the Association, Andrew McFarland, medical superintendent of the Illinois State Hospital, read a paper on "Minor Mental Maladies," which stimulated substantial discussion on the issue of intellectual involvement in insanity. Gray, of course, remained unalterably opposed to any form of partial insanity: "Insanity is something more than the perturbed emotions and the loss of self-control." He then asserted that disturbance of the moral feelings led ultimately to dementia, "the terminal stage of insanity." John Tyler, of the McLean Asylum, challenged him on the question of melancholia:

I wish to know whether Dr. Gray has any doubt that the starting point [of melancholia] is in the feelings, and not in the perversion of thought?
*Dr. Gray:* I presume that in melancholia the feelings are the first affected, and that before the intellect is perceptibly involved, it is a disease.
*Dr. Tyler:* But would you call it insanity?
*Dr. Gray:* I should call it a simple form of melancholia. I should not call it a case of moral insanity, as represented in medical works.
*Dr. Tyler:* But would you call it a case of insanity at all, until the intellect was somewhat affected?
*Dr. Gray:* I should not until the person began to lose self-control. A case of simple morbid feelings, of depressed spirits, of wretchedness, or unhappiness, I should not consider a case of insanity.

At this point, Isaac Ray joined the discussion: "If I understand the inference rightly, it was that we had no right to call any case of mental disturbance insanity, unless we could show intellectual aberration. Well, there are cases—call them what you please; the name will not change the thing."[3]

Gray's circular argument on the relationship between reason and self-control was typical of those who believed that the mind was unitary. Although he asserted that insanity was more than "perturbed emotions and the loss of self-control," he identified the loss of self-control as the first symptom of intellectual involvement in an emotional insanity, melancholia. Ray appealed to empiricism; the cases were there to be observed, "call them what you please." Nevertheless, the moral somaticists rejected the concept of partial insanity either on religious grounds or on the ground that it smacked of phrenology, which by the 1860s had fallen into disrepute.

Bucknill and Tuke did not take any radical new position relative to the partial insanities. Their thought represented the strict organic psychiatry that was flourishing at the time among the Germans, notably Wilhelm Griesinger. Bucknill and Tuke believed that mental diseases could originate in an individual faculty or propensity, but they equivocated on the issue of whether or not the intellect could remain intact in cases of partial insanity.[4]

## Emotional Insanity: Moral Insanity and Homicidal Impulse

By the mid-1850s, Prichard's original conception of moral insanity had become muddled and misunderstood. Alienists held a variety of theoretical positions: the moral somaticists rejected the existence of emotional insanity altogether, though some saw moral insanity as a condition in which the derangement of the emotions was secondary to a fundamental intellectual derangement; others believed that emotional derangement was the first sign of a form of insanity that would progress to frank involvement of the intellect, delusions, and dementia. Finally, there were those who accepted Prichard's original conception, that the emotions could indeed be deranged while the intellect and the will remained intact. Lawyers raised the moral insanity defense in a wide variety of medico-legal circumstances. As John Ordronaux, one of the most prominent medical jurisprudents of the period remarked: "Satan himself becomes converted into a simple moral lunatic."[5]

## Moral Insanity Challenged

Clearly, the concept of moral insanity threatened the ideas and values as well as the medical judgments of a large number of physicians. Like Ordronaux, W. S. Chipley, superintendent of the Eastern Kentucky Asylum, believed that moral insanity was a chimera and that other cases of insanity and depravity were so designated. He suggested: "Of all the cases adduced as instances of moral insanity the homicidal variety is the most important." He went on to list four misconceptions:

1st. Such as are not insane, who shed the blood of their fellow-creatures under the influence of passions that have known no restraints. [Chipley maintained that it was the duty of men to control their passions.]
2nd . . . the subjects of impulse to do wrong, without motive. [Chipley interpreted:] I do not believe that every impulse of this kind makes a man a maniac. The intellect was still sound . . . .
3rd . . . instances of moral insanity in which the intellectual impairment was indisputable . . . the grossest delusions. [Here Chipley called delusional or homicidal insanity moral insanity because the result was immoral.]
4th. The fourth class embraces those unfortunate subjects in whom there is no apparent delusion, but the details of whose history warrant the inference that their understanding is unsound. Well marked physical symptoms proved the existence of disease affecting the brain, and his paroxysms of fury showed a paralysis of the ruling powers of the mind.[6]

Chipley cited other medical superintendents to support his opinion: "Dr. McFarland [Illinois State Hospital] has under care nearly 3,000 insane persons, and has failed to find a single case of what is termed moral insanity . . . Dr. Gray in 5,000 observations; Dr. Workman [Provincial Lunatic Asylum, Toronto, Canada] 2,000; the late Dr. Ranney, [New York City Lunatic Asylum, Blackwell's Island], 6,000; to which I add my own observation during the last eleven years." Chipley credited, or blamed, the courts' acceptance of the doctrine upon the scholarship of Isaac Ray's *Medical Jurisprudence of Insanity*.

The absence of any apparent motive in a homicide often raised the question of moral insanity. In 1866 John Curwen, medical superintendent of the Pennsylvania State Lunatic Hospital, was summoned to the office of the secretary of the commonwealth for consultation in the case of a Mrs. Grinder, of Pittsburgh. She had been found guilty of poisoning her neighbors. The apparent lack of motive led some physicians of standing and some members of the legislature to believe that she was insane and ought not to be executed.

Curwen investigated the case and concluded that he had found a clear motive: the theft of some money that Mrs. Grinder knew was in the house. He also discovered other murders she had committed for theft or deception, including that of an infant. He asserted, "The evidence was clear that she had been a bad woman her whole life; there was not a trace of insanity about her. The only thing that looked at all like insanity was the fact that she was sometimes hysterical at her catamenial periods."[7]

Dain noted that objections to the concept of moral insanity were raised on theoretical, ethical, and religious grounds, but he suggested that the principal arguments were ethical and religious ones. Alienists were concerned about the effects upon society if the depraved were excused from the consequences of their behavior. Dain maintains that much of the disagreement was clearly nonmedical and that the validity of moral insanity as a medical entity was not a predominant issue.[8] Although it is true that some alienists rejected a primary derangement of the moral faculties on religious grounds, all objections to the existence of such a phenomenon were not reducible to belief.

The central theoretical issue in the moral insanity question was whether or not the boundary between malevolence and malady could be demonstrated empirically. Some of the alienists who rejected moral insanity as acquired disease of the moral faculty did not reject instances of moral imbecility, conceived of either as the underdevelopment of the moral sense in mentally defective persons or as the inability to reason correctly on moral questions because of inadequate intelligence. This group also accepted instances of moral insanity, so-called, when a well-defined delusion motivated the immoral conduct. These formulations left unanswered the question of whether or not a person who was unable to reason correctly on moral issues was morally insane, or, if so, how was such a condition to be demonstrated empirically. What critical features of such cases could separate the person unable to reason correctly on moral issues from the person who chose not to reason correctly?

### The Townley Case

The celebrated case of George Victor Townley illuminates a number of themes in the social and legal history of psychiatry, but the divergent opinions held by the alienists in this instance reflect the obstinate question of the role of intellect in moral reasoning and conduct. In the final analysis, neither the British legal system nor British alienists answered the question of whether Townley's defect in reasoning was feigned insanity, evidence of a diseased intellect, a diseased moral faculty, or depravity.

The essential details of the case are as follows: when Townley's fiancée, a Miss Goodwin, asked to be released from a protracted engagement in order to marry another man, Townley arranged for a final meeting with her, at which he stabbed her fatally. He had planned the meeting for such purpose, and afterward he made no effort to conceal the crime or to escape arrest—behaviors that had been identified in 1838 by Ray as signs of insane homicide.[9]

The testimony in favor of Townley's insanity rested upon the evidence of Forbes Winslow, who examined him on two occasions, on November 18 for two hours and again on December 10 for three quarters of an hour. Winslow believed that he was insane because of his lack of remorse and his belief that he had the right to kill his fiancée if he chose to. Winslow regarded these statements as evidence of a diseased intellect; he "seemed incapable of reasoning correctly on any moral subject." Winslow diagnosed Townley's belief in the conspiracy as delusional: "There were six conspirators plotting against him with a view to destroy him, with a chief conspirator at their head. This conspiracy was still going on while he was in prison, and he had no doubt that if he was at liberty, they would continue their operations against him, and in order to escape their evil purposes he would have to leave the country." The Commissioners in Lunacy, however, interpreted what Winslow diagnosed as delusion as a natural belief justified by the facts.[10] Miss Goodwin had, in fact, been advised by family and friends to break off the engagement because of Townley's want of means and settled employment.

Winslow believed that the man was morally insane because of his inability to reason correctly on any moral subject, a finding separate from the supposed delusion. Winslow based his diagnosis upon the murderer's claim that he was free to kill the woman if he chose to, and upon the finding that an aunt had committed suicide, which alienists in 1864 considered "hereditary taint."

Even though the jury returned the verdict of willful murder, doubt about Townley's sanity was sufficient enough so that the judge asked the Home Secretary to send the Commissioners in Lunacy to make an evaluation of the man's condition. Although the commissioners believed that he had been justly convicted according to English law, they did not consider him to be of sound mind "in view of the extravagant opinions deliberately professed by him, of his extraordinarily perverted moral sense, and of hereditary taint."[11]

Other prominent British alienists disagreed with Winslow's assessment of Townley. Henry Maudsley and C. Lockhard-Robinson, the editors of the *Journal of Mental Science*, wrote a monograph analyzing the case in terms of the three possible categories of partial insanity that would have identified the murderer as a dangerous lunatic: delusional insanity (monomania), moral insanity, and impulsive insanity.

The editors rejected outright the existence of a delusion. They suggested that Townley had duped Winslow. They did not regard his claim that he was free to kill Miss Goodwin as evidence of delusion. "Such reasoning may argue moral perversion," they said, "but there is no evidence in it of intellectual disorder."[12]

Winslow believed that Townley's extravagant opinions on moral issues were evidence of moral insanity. The editors rejected this diagnosis because they believed that the empirical evidence of moral insanity was a clearly defined hereditary taint. In Townley's case, "the utmost that could be said in favour of hereditary insanity was . . . that a grand-aunt had committed suicide, and some more distant relatives had been insane. No linear ancestor of the prisoner was said to have been insane." Not only did the theory of moral insanity not explain every circumstance of the case, in Maudsley's and Robinson's opinion, but also it was positively incompatible with certain of the circumstances. They made a clear theoretical distinction between moral insanity and moral perversion, "which the birch-rod marvelously improves."[13]

Maudsley and Robinson concluded that Townley was not insane. Bucknill examined him on two occasions while he was under observation at Bethlem and also concluded that he was sane. Yet, in the uncertainty surrounding the case, his death sentence was commuted to penal servitude for life. He very soon after committed suicide. Because the issues were clearly laid out, this case for years was exemplary on both sides of the Atlantic.

### Homicidal Impulse

The homicidal impulse was another form of insanity that alienists believed had its primary locus in the emotions. In this condition, the lunatic felt the urge to kill someone, but at the same time understood that this was an immoral and hideous crime.

Most alienists followed Pinel and Esquirol in their identification of *manie sans délire*, or homicidal monomania. In the United States, the condition came to be called the "homicidal impulse," and those who accepted the reality of such a condition indeed deemed it a predictor of dangerousness. Prichard believed in the primacy of the homicidal impulse and contended that a defect in reason, the delusion, was a "secondary thought or mere accessory to the engrossing impulse."[14] Tuke agreed with Prichard that the genesis of the homicidal impulse was in the propensities rather than in the reason.[15]

Gray rejected the idea of homicidal impulse because he believed that, so long as the intellect was intact, lunatics were capable of controlling their behavior and were therefore not insane. However, he was not clear in his theoretical position on the question of behavioral control. He maintained that insanity was more than perturbed emotions and the loss of self-control, but, if well-defined physical disease were present, or if the homicidal impulse had been preceded by an identifiable change in character, then he took these findings to be evidence of brain disease. He accepted the possibility of such a form of insanity within the context of his own somatic theories, but he rejected the idea that homicidal impulse could exist without physical disease on religious grounds.

Samuel B. Woodward reported such a case of homicidal impulse in 1845. A young man consulted him because he had become obsessed with an extraordinary desire to kill. He concealed his feelings from his family and friends, and the idea gradually subsided. But then, in the course of setting up a business with his brother-in-law, he was seized again with the desire to kill him. So strong was this impulse that he left his work without notice and went to his father's house. Once again, the young man summoned Woodward, who prescribed some remedies and a diet, but did not commit him to the asylum. Woodward believed that such cases were rare, but he did not doubt their existence: "That active impulses affect the mind of man, under some circumstances, quite controllable, disconnected entirely with any existing delusion, cannot be doubted."[16] He ended the report by saying that he hoped that the patient had recovered, but that he had not heard from him again.

### Volitional Insanity: *Mania Transitoria* and Epilepsy

Early in the 1850s, a new theoretical concept, *mania transitoria*, emerged. In 1851 the French alienist Castelnau reported a case of an apparently healthy person who was seized with an attack of mania that ran a brief course and then passed away, leaving the patient completely recovered. In an 1863 paper in the *Journal of Mental Science*, Henry Maudsley explored the concept and suggested its connection with epilepsy. Castelnau's original conception, however, posited the existence of a phenomenon that was supposed to arise in the absolute absence of any pre-existing brain disease. *Mania transitoria* could, but did not necessarily, take the homicidal form.[17]

From the outset, the existence of *mania transitoria* gave rise to considerable medico-legal doubt. An authentic *mania transitoria* exhibited three elements: a sudden onset, a short duration in terms of hours or days, and complete recovery without sequellae. The patient was insensible during the attack and amnesic after recovery. *Mania transitoria* was characterized by excessive destructiveness. Many cases in the medical literature were characterized by one or two of these elements, particularly excessive destructiveness in some of the homicides credited to lunatics. In medico-legal cases, the insanity defense was occasionally raised using *mania transitoria*, but typically only one or two of its characteristics could be identified in the final analysis.

### The Case of Dr. Wright

John P. Gray reported such a case in 1864. David M. Wright, a Norfolk, Virginia, white physician murdered a black army officer, a lieutenant named Sandborn. Wright pleaded insanity, claiming he had experienced a transient psychosis. The lieutenant had marched a company of black troops through the main streets of the city on the day of the homicide. Wright became upset by this news when he was informed of it by his family. Although he did nothing immediately, he later accosted the officer and shot him. President Lincoln summoned Gray to examine Wright.[18]

Because Gray had rejected the theoretical possibility of *mania transitoria*, he examined Wright for other evidence of pre-existing disease. Spending more than two hours with the man and reviewing all the testimony given at the hearing, he found that Wright was in satisfactory physical health; and even though he had always written eccentric medical prescriptions, no explicit changes in his behavior or his character had occurred during the past five years. Gray did not find clinically significant the fact that Wright had received the news of the defeat at Gettysburg but had not learned the fate of his son, who was in the battle. Gray noted that Wright exhibited no greater depression than was natural under such circumstances and found no evidence of latent insanity or physical pathology. He concluded that a burst of passion is not the same as an uncontrollable impulse. He testified that latent insanity, indeed, could emerge in an act of violence, but that it did not "instantly disappear with the accomplishment of the violent act, as it has done, if it existed, in the present instance."[19] Gray concluded, therefore, that *mania transitoria* was a chimera.

By contrast, at the Association meeting in June 1865, Isaac Ray read a paper on *mania transitoria*, citing the case of Bernard Clangley, reported in the *Belfast* (Ireland) *Journal* on March 4, 1864. Clangley was a guest in the home of Peter Reilly and his wife. He arose during the night and stabbed his host. He did not conceal his actions and went immediately to the police to turn himself in. No motive for the homicide was elicited. Although no medical witness who may have been conversant with the concept of *mania transitoria* was called to testify, the court applied the McNaugten rule and Clangley was found guilty.[20]

Ray accepted the existence of *mania transitoria*: "There can scarcely be a reasonable doubt that Clangley committed the bloody act in a short and sudden paroxysm of mania. . . . The occurrence of the homicide shortly after going to sleep, would naturally raise the suspicion that Clangley was in a state of somnolentia, or sleep-drunkenness, as the Germans call it. . . . In this state of mental confusion and alarm, he mistakes the first person who comes within reach for his imaginary foe, and attacks him with whatever weapon comes to hand."[21] However, evidence that Clangley's was a case of somnolentia was lacking; it was theoretical speculation that Ray applied to the case.

Ray's paper generated a lively discussion. Clement A. Walker related a case of Charles H. Steadman's. A woman killed her child with a hammer in the presence of her sister, suddenly and without any warning. She maintained a perfect rational conception of her guilt, her explanation for killing the child having been: "I thought the wall opened and I saw my child lying out in the cold, and crying for bread."[22]

G. S. C. Choate, superintendent of the Lunatic Hospital at Taunton, Massachusetts, said that it was "dangerous to accept any theory which would lead them to admit that a person never known to have been insane should commit a crime under sudden impulse."[23] Several other alienists present at the discussion contributed cases that supported the existence of *mania transitoria*, and consensus was reached that it was not connected with any specific prodromata and thereby impossible to predict. There was general agreement, however, that masturbation could precipitate the attack.

The idea of *mania transitoria* was a logical extension of the concept of moral somaticism. Alienists conceived of the brain as subject to the same biological forces and processes as any other visceral organ. It followed, then, that it could exhibit a state akin to spasms and reflexes in the viscera. Those who rejected the idea did so on the assumption that a disease without a history was a contradiction in terms. Both the acceptance and the rejection of the theory was, in the final analysis, founded upon moral somaticism.

### Epilepsy and Epileptic Insanity

In the early 1860s, *mania transitoria* became linked with epilepsy. Alienists recognized that epilepsy was complicated by dementia from repeated seizures in some cases, but certainly not in all. But also associated with epilepsy was a peculiarly dangerous form of mania. The British alienist George Mann Burrows had described it in 1828. He posited the idea that seizure activity not terminating in a *grand mal* seizure "acts on the brain in a peculiar mode, and imparts to it that particular action denominated epileptic mania." Epileptics were credited with the potential for the most grisly acts of violence.[24]

For those who rejected the idea of an idiopathic *mania transitoria*, the connection of such episodes of mania with epilepsy was entirely logical. According to the British alienist Henry Maudsley, writing in 1868, "a *furor transitorious* lasting a few hours or days, and accompanied by vivid hallucinations and destructive tendencies" had been observed by so many clinicians that it was impossible to doubt its occurrence. Yet, of the existence of *mania transitoria* in its idiopathic form, Maudsley remarked wryly, "Since the time of Esquirol there had been in France an ambition to discover a new variety of insanity, and to coin a new name for it; but the verbal distinctions had not often stood the test of exact observation."[25]

Epileptic lunatics who were committed to asylums were regarded as unpredictable, usually violent, and a bad influence on the sensibilities of the ordinary insane. There was agitation for separate asylums for epileptics. Alienists tried a variety of sedatives and other drugs to modify the frequency and severity of the fits as well as the general violence surrounding the presence of the epileptic in the asylum.[26]

### The Winnemore Case

In 1867 Ray reported the case of George Winnemore, which illustrates the early stage in the beliefs about the relationship between epilepsy and homicidal insanity. On April 25, 1867, Winnemore was accused of having cut the throat of a woman named Dorcus Magilton and was brought to trial within the week. The court-appointed counsel did not have adequate time to prepare the case, but, because of Winnemore's epilepsy, the insanity defense was set up.

During the course of the trial, several physicians were called upon to testify, but only one was an alienist. According to Isaac Ray, "Their testimony was confined to some desultory remarks respecting the effect of epilepsy on the mind, but it embraced nothing like a complete methodical statement of facts. . . . No medical witness had made a particular examination of the prisoner."[27] The counsel believed that the trial had not been fair, but the effort to obtain a new one failed. An attempt to have the governor appoint a lunacy commission to investigate the prisoner's mental condition also failed. As a last resort, a few days before the execution, counsel requested that some medical men who were familiar with epilepsy interview Winnemore.

Isaac Ray, J. H. Worthington, superintendent of Friends' Asylum, and S. Preston Jones, assistant physician at the Pennsylvania Hospital for the Insane, visited Winnemore in jail. Ray and his colleagues elicited a history of *petit mal* seizures from early childhood, as many as several a day to as few as twelve a month. The seizures were followed by varying periods of retrograde amnesia. Ray suggested that the shock of finding his friend with her throat slashed precipitated a *petit mal* seizure characterized by a period of unconsciousness and retrograde amnesia. But Winnemore claimed a perfect recollection of having gone to call upon the victim and finding her dead. Ray alternately suggested that Winnemore had suffered a *petit mal* seizure and was unconscious when he committed the deed.[28]

The alienists addressed a petition to the governor of Pennsylvania but it was refused. Winnemore was excuted on August 29, just four months after the homicide. He insisted to the last that he had not committed the deed.

### From Static to Dynamic Neurophysiology

The idea of *mania transitoria* and its possible causes in the visceral physiology and in epilepsy reflected a change in the understanding of the neurophysiological basis for insanity. Partial insanity and phrenology supported a conception of the brain as a collection of anatomical loci with individual physiologies, mutually exclusive and static. Alienists who rejected the existence of the partial insanities explained these phenomena as early manifestations of progressive disease. Insanity progressed, they believed, to its terminus, dementia. Still, this conception reflected a static neurophysiology.

The change from a static to a dynamic neurophysiology followed the work of Griesinger, his student Theodor Meynert, and other advocates of German mechanistic psychiatry. The concept of a physiological unconscious was reinforced by Meynert's elucidation of association pathways and his conception of the hierarchical structure of the brain. Thus, consciousness was located in the higher cortical centers; the unconscious in the lower, or supporting, structures.[29] The use of the terms subconscious (literally "under") and unconscious in the English language medical literature from 1860 to after the turn of the twentieth century generally meant a physiological unconscious.[30]

By 1860 Henry Maudsley was an influential British alienist,

jurisprudent, and pedagogue. He embraced the German program for scientific medicine and believed that the advance of psychological medicine was best achieved through laboratory research. He eschewed a metaphysical approach to psychiatry, and, though his physiology was entirely derivative, he posited a strict mechanical physiology for insanity. He published a textbook on the subject in 1867, immediately revised parts of it, and published a second edition in 1868 in order to remove some obscurities and to emphasize the physiological over the metaphysical study of mental phenomena.[31]

Maudsley conceived of the brain as a physiological unity. Any dysfunction rendered the whole organ unstable and the lunatic unpredictable. Dangerousness, therefore, became a feature of the intensity of the dysfunction rather than the form. All types of lunacy could make the patient dangerous.

Maudsley proposed yet another classification and nomenclature for insanity. He theorized that the affective disorder was the fundamental fact of insanity and the intellectual disorder was of the second order. "To insist upon delusion as a criterion of insanity," he wrote, "is to ignore some of the gravest and most dangerous forms of mental disease."[32]

Maudsley, like Winslow, Bucknill, Tuke, and others, was unwilling to propose the absolute absence of any intellectual morbidity in moral insanity. Because affect was more fundamental than cognition, it followed that intellectual activity could not be left entirely unaffected by morbid feelings. If the lunatic were affected with moral insanity, it was likely to pass into intellectual disorder and dementia. The morally insane lunatic was dangerous because, left to his own devices or placed under conditions of excitement, the "unconscious life appears to get mastery, and drives him to immoral, extravagant, and dangerous acts." By the "unconscious life" Maudsley meant the energy produced at the neurophysiological level, not the dynamic unconscious.[33]

Similarly, Maudsley maintained that a single morbid idea, or delusion, could not exist in an otherwise sound mind: "In vain do men pretend that the mind of the monomaniac is sound apart from his delusion." He believed that the delusion was a symptom of a fundamental disorder in the physiological integrity of the mind and that its effects were global. It predisposed lunatics to "conclusive mental phenomena," thereby making them decidedly unstable and predictably dangerous. Unlike Bucknill and Tuke, who maintained that the content of the delusion was the predictor of dangerousness, Maudsley reasoned that "the morbid centre reacts injuriously on the neighbouring centres, and there is no guarantee that at any moment the most desperate consequences may not ensue." Sometimes a discoverable relationship existed between an act of violence and the delusion, but at other times none could be discovered, nor was it necessary, in Maudsley's opinion, to seek such a relationship. The existence of the delusion merely indicated the unstable state of the brain tissue. The lunatic laboring under a delusion, no matter how benign its contents may appear, was predictably dangerous.[34]

During this entire period, 1840–70, the somatic model of insanity predominated. That insanity was a disease of the brain was never seriously questioned, though alienists held a wide variety of opinions about the etiological effect of deranged visceral organs and nonphysical, or "moral," causes of brain pathology. During the 1860s, the conception of the brain as a collection of static anatomical loci changed to a view of it as a neurodynamic organ. Maudsley's 1868 textbook exemplified this change; he imagined that the brain in insanity was friable, unstable, and liable to instantaneous disequilibrium. The practical result of this change was that all insane people were believed to be highly unpredictable and possibly dangerous.

# The Non-Asylum Treatment of    5
the Insane

Over the next four decades, 1870–1910, social and scientific changes transformed the practice of psychiatry from mere superintendency of the insane to active medical care; asylums into hospitals; and superintendents into a regular medical specialty. Improved histopathological techniques and modest advancements in chemistry, chiefly in Germany, turned attention away from interest in the moral causes of insanity toward an intensified search for physical lesions in the pathology laboratory. Reinforced by discoveries in medical bacteriology, by 1870 alienists did not question the assumption that insanity was physical disease of the brain. It was believed that the condition was hereditary; B. A. Morel's degeneracy theory and Lamarckian ideas about the transmission of acquired characteristics enhanced belief in the transmission of an imperfect nervous system from generation to generation, but added the feature of atavism to the overall theory.[1]

The major impetus for both intellectual and practical changes came from the new specialty of neurology. The medical superintendents and neurologists did not differ essentially in their beliefs about the nature of insanity, but the neurologists challenged all facets of the asylum system.[2] At this time, the 1870s, both groups generally accepted the idea that insanity was a physiological derangement of the nervous system brought about by both physical and moral causes. The real difference of opinion centered about the clinical manifestations of the disease and how best it should be treated. The principal concern of the neurologists was the quasi-judicial power of asylum superintendents. Neurologists favored extra-asylum treatment of the insane and began to collect handsome fees for it.

### Dangerousness and Involuntary Commitment

By 1870 public distrust of mental hospitals had led to a substantial amount of legislation designed to protect sane people from involuntary commitment.[3] These laws differed materially as to the procedure for commitment and the role played by medical superintendents or general physicians. Most of the laws, however, maintained the principle that the state had the right and the responsibility to treat the insane. In New York, for example, the person had to be "insane, and so far disordered in his senses, as to endanger his own person, and the persons and property of others if permitted to go at large."[4] Although the New York law specifically exempted cases of chronic and harmless insanity, it allowed for lunatics to be admitted for their own welfare. The law did not define "harmless," but, because lack of treatment constituted a danger to the individual, few cases were regarded as harmless in the final analysis.[5] Alienists also believed that any type of lunatic could become dangerous at any moment. Richard W. Fox pointed out in his study of involuntary commitment in California between 1870 and 1930 that practitioners generally believed that small crimes could lead to larger crimes.[6]

In both the United States and Great Britain, physicians believed that insanity and danger were inseparable. In Great Britain, public agitation that sane people were being involuntarily committed to asylums prompted the House of Commons to appoint a committee in 1877 to investigate the lunacy laws. Although the belief that early confinement offered the best hope for cure still prevailed, the lunacy law of Great Britain, as it turned out, was formulated without regard for the therapeutic welfare of the insane.[7]

Bucknill believed that the concept of dangerousness went beyond the legal definition, namely, "to inflict physical, not moral injury." He also maintained that "harmless" was not necessarily the opposite of "dangerous": "In the springtime of the common law a great lawyer or doctor who had become insane might not be dangerous if he were not violent; but such a man at the present day, who went about town babbling, not of green fields but of family secrets, would certainly not be harmless."[8]

Whenever the issue of involuntary commitment arose, physicians referred to both the importance of early treatment and to the danger they believed was associated with insanity. At the twenty-ninth annual meeting of the American Medical Association at Buffalo, June 4, 1878, the proceedings reflected substantial interest in this issue. At that meeting, the Association adopted a set of resolutions which documented the predominant position that involuntary commitment was a therapeutic necessity. Members asserted that the resolutions were formulated from a strictly medical standpoint and were "a deliberate declaration, by the representative body of the medical profession of the United States." The resolutions declared:

*First.* That insanity is a disease; and
*Second.* That personal restraint is an essential element of its therapeutic treatment.
*Third.* They also concisely state the distinction between the medical and police cases of restraint.
*Fourth.* They declare that proof of insanity justifies the therapeutical restraint of the insane person, with a view to his cure, just as fully as proof of his dangerous conduct justifies that police restraint which is intended to prevent injury.[9]

In practice, however, physicians did not make such a distinction between therapeutic and police restraint because they believed that any lunatic was potentially dangerous.

Medical superintendents and neurologists disagreed little upon the issue of restraint of dangerous types. What did create controversy was the neurologists' declaration that fewer of them were dangerous than alienists believed. In 1879 William A. Hammond, a leading New York neurologist and critic of the medical superintendents, addressed the Medical Society of New York on the subject "The Non-Asylum Treatment of the Insane." His theme was that "in many cases sequestration is not only unnecessary but positively injurious." He touted the superiority of the family-care system. Yet, when the issue of dangerousness arose, he distinguished between mild cases of insanity and the troublesome or dangerous. All those who refused food and exhibited homicidal/suicidal tendencies or delusions/morbid impulses that prompted them to the destruction of property or to other acts of violence should be sequestered.[10] Hammond suggested that the "best form of sequestration" was to lock the lunatic in the physician's house. The poor, on the other hand, would be sent to the asylum.

### Professional Ideology of Involuntary Treatment

Physicians believed that, if dangerousness were the sole criterion for involuntary commitment, then the nondangerous insane were left without protection. John Ordronaux, for forty-eight years a professor of medical jurisprudence at various prominent schools of law and medicine as well as the first New York State Commissioner in Lunacy, maintained that the spirit of the New York state lunacy law was to protect the insane, though the protection envisioned by the alienists was of quite a different character from that advocated by the neurologists and a reform group associated with them, the National Association for the Protection of the Insane. Ordronaux reasoned that, if only the furiously mad could be legally confined, then the law would fail to "protect a large proportion of the insane in every community, and the most helpless class would receive neither recognition nor protection, no hospitals or asylums would be open to them."[11] Although Ordronaux believed that the dangerous and the nondangerous insane could be separated in principle, alienists had not yet established a method in the asylum system to do so.

Nonmedical organizations also concerned themselves with the involuntary commitment of the insane. At the National Conference of Charities, held at Buffalo, New York, June 7, 1888, Stephen Smith, who succeeded Ordronaux as Commissioner in Lunacy in 1882, chaired a special committee on the Commitment and Detention of the Insane. Smith reported that the committee had not agreed upon all the propositions, but he published those formulations upon which there had been general agreement, namely, that the state had the right to deprive the insane of their personal liberty when they were violent, threatening violence, wandering at large, or the disease required treatment. But Smith also believed that not all the insane should be involuntarily committed; the harmless who were being cared for adequately by their families or friends required mere overseeing to assure that they were adequately protected.[12]

The practical result of public interest in the commitment of the insane was that these assertions resulted in more commitments than fewer owing to the various conceptions of dangerousness held by physicians, lawyers, humanitarian reformers, and the public at large. The rhetoric of the public interest groups tended to reflect an understanding of homicidal insanity as an easily diagnosed condition which remained static and a belief that the dangerous insane could be readily identified and separated from the harmless. Medical thinkers, on the other hand, particularly practicing medical superintendents, contended that dangerousness was a potential in all lunatics because of the unstable condition of the brain.[13]

### The Newcomer Case

In the final analysis, the standard of dangerousness and the legal doctrine of *parens patriae* were inseparable. For example, in 1877 Mrs. Nancy J. Newcomer sued E. H. van Deusen, of the Kalamazoo (Michigan) Asylum for the Insane, "for trespass, false imprisonment and malpractice." Her records showed conclusively that she was insane when committed. The alienist Henry Hurd maintained that "the judge charged that it was a fundamental principle of law that *no person* may be deprived of liberty . . . without due process of law, and that any involuntary control or seclusion of another against his will, is imprisonment. . . . In other words, any detention of a person . . . unless actually dangerous, is false imprisonment."[14] Because the court could find no evidence that Mrs. Newcomer was dangerous before she was brought to the asylum by her daughter or during her sojourn there, the jury awarded her $6,000 damages.

Van Deusen appealed to the state supreme court on the basis that a hospital was not a prison and that it was a natural right to restrain the insane, not dependent upon any statute for validity. The court, granting a new trial, reversed the decision on the basis that: (1) Insanity was a disease, and the essential element in treatment was restraint of personal liberty; (2) Restraint was not by police power to prevent danger, but by humanity for treatment; and (3) The office of medical superintendent was quasi-judicial in character, and he could legally decide when individuals could be confined or discharged. Although Mrs. Newcomer's potential dangerousness was central to the decision of the lower court, the Supreme Court reversed the decision on the doctrine of *parens patriae*.[15]

Although nonmedical thinkers felt that the dangerous and the harmless insane could be readily separated, physicians maintained that dangerousness was difficult to predict, even after a protracted observation in the asylum. During the parliamentary inquiry of 1877, Lord Shaftesbury, the prime mover in bringing about lunacy law reform and for fifty years a Commissioner in Lunacy, testified in favor of commitment for observation in all cases of insanity. He stated that he could not recall a single instance in his long experience of a false commitment. As part of his testimony, he presented statistics compiled at his request by William Orange, medical superintendent of London's Broadmoor Asylum. These statistics showed that in 147 of 326 cases of homicidal insanity, the illness was recognized before the overt act was committed. In 78 of these cases, the lunatic was believed to be harmless. Lord Shaftesbury also expressed the opinion that too many discharges were being made before adequate recovery.[16]

## When to Discharge, If to Discharge

Medical superintendents recognized the difficulty of predicting dangerousness within the context of assessing recovery. Both American and British physicians agreed that early commitment was advisable because dangerousness was difficult to predict, but they differed in their opinion about discharges. Lord Shaftesbury referred to the common practice among British alienists to furlough or to discharge outright those who were recovering. At the Association meetings throughout the 1870s, American medical superintendents discussed the question of recovery and how it could be assessed. There was general agreement that recovered lunatics were free of delusions and could control their behavior. Although the letter was relatively easy to assess, a lunatic could easily conceal delusions, an observation already widely reported in the medical literature.

At the Association meeting held at Auburn, New York, in 1875, the issue of furlough to relieve overcrowding arose within the context of a discussion of recovery after protracted periods of lunacy. Although alienists were convinced by this time that cases lasting for more than one year were hopeless, several of them reported unusual recoveries, thus raising the possibility of cure where none had been expected. Robert F. Baldwin, of the Western Lunatic Asylum in Staunton, Virginia, reported that the practice of furloughing both chronic and recovering lunatics had been initiated by Francis S. Stribling, his predecessor, and that it had been continued with success. Bucknill, who was invited to participate in the discussions at this meeting, reported that furloughing was common practice in English asylums. He said that he routinely sent recovering patients to the seaside or to reside with friends, including those who had been violent during the acute illness. Bucknill contended that violent patients should be given trial furloughs and that "in dealing with lunatics, some risks must be run and borne."[17]

Several medical superintendents disagreed with Bucknill that such risk should be taken. Thomas S. Kirkbride arose to dissent. He said that early in his career he was disposed to give maximum liberty to all patients, but that experience had made him more cautious. He did not believe that recovery could be assessed adequately to take the risk of ever releasing a dangerous or suicidal lunatic. Of the positive reports of other medical superintendents, he said, "This discussion has impressed me very strongly with the danger of making general rules from an observation of a limited number of cases."[18] He added that, even if patients demonstrated no dangerous propensities, those who were half cured often did not improve and relapsed when they were furloughed. He rejected *a priori* that any patient, whether dangerous or harmless, could ever be pronounced cured with certainty.

Other medical superintendents joined Kirkbride in expressing reservations about the practice of furloughing. Eugene Grissom, superintendent of the Insane Asylum for North Carolina, arose to relate his experience. He reported three cases of homicide and suicide committed by discharged patients who had been considered dangerous. One of these, "having been at home only a short time . . . destroyed his father, wife and two children during the same paroxysm."[19]

Despite this firm rejection of the idea of furlough by influential members of the Association, the younger physicians, Baldwin, Henry Landor, medical superintendent of the London (Ontario) Asylum, and D. R. Wallace, of the Hospital for the Insane, Austin, Texas, pursued the issue at the 1876 meeting. These medical superintendents maintained that: (1) Asylums were unnecessarily overcrowded with convalescent and chronic patients; (2) Patients of both classes could be paroled with minimal risk to the public; and (3) Such patients would be better off outside the asylum. The superintendents believed that recovery, or chronicity, in some cases, could be assessed with an acceptable degree of accuracy, and, if patients did relapse, they could be returned to the asylum.

Wallace described his experience within the context of his routine progress report to the Association at large. He presented seven cases in which furloughing had been successful. He believed that the alienist was able to predict dangerousness or the absence of it, though he did not suggest a particular method.[20]

Landor undertook an experiment to test the hypothesis. The results of his study were published in the 1876 *American Journal of Insanity*.[21] Of the 114 lunatics studied, 37 were "explicitly dangerous." Although 5 of this latter group relapsed while on leave and had to be returned to the asylum, 2 ultimately improved enough to be discharged. One of these individuals, a case of homicidal mania according to Landor, relapsed because of "insufficient food and hard work. Afterwards [he was] discharged cured and has been well for two years."

Baldwin also believed that insane homicide could be predicted. He, too, read a paper before the Association in which he described his experience with furloughing fifty patients to family and friends. He assessed each of them in terms of their behavior within the asylum and of the environment to which they were to be returned. Baldwin saw furlough as a therapeutic measure and felt that he had hastened recoveries.[22]

A. E. MacDonald rejected the validity of Baldwin's findings. Like Kirkbride, speaking against drawing any scientific conclusions from so small a sample of cases, he regarded both Landor's and Baldwin's cases as exceptions. Referring to Baldwin's results, MacDonald did not believe that the two suicides in fifty cases of furloughing justified the experiment: "Had all the cases been improved by the furloughing, (which I do not think was shown,) to my thinking the evil result in these two cases would outweigh the benefit obtained in the others."[23]

Kirkbride also maintained his conservative position. In these cases, too, he believed that the patients were exceptions from which no generalizations could be drawn. He rejected the idea that the mentally ill could be made worse by being in the asylum. But his principal reason for rejecting the idea of furlough was his belief that dangerousness was a critical feature of all insanity. He reiterated his position by saying, "More persons lost their lives and were injured by insane persons being at large than by all the railroad accidents that occurred during the same period."[24]

Notwithstanding the fearful case reports and the authority of Kirkbride, others cited cases with positive results and the overall consensus seemed to favor cautious experimentation and furloughing. Others who sided with Kirkbride gave evidence that dangerousness was often a feature of those laboring under concealed delusions and that the most dangerous lunatics often appeared quiet and harmless. Limited experiments with furloughing continued to be reported in the annual reports of the asylums and at the Association meetings. Because of the general lack of confidence in the assessment of cure, however, and the prevailing idea that the insane could at any instant become dangerous, the practice was never adopted as a major program to relieve the overcrowded asylums.

### Failure of Extra-Asylum Care

Medical superintendents' belief that most lunatics were unpredictable and dangerous delayed the process of providing alternative settings for care, particularly receiving wards in general hospitals and urban psychopathic hospitals. Toward the turn of the century, some receiving facilities were organized, particularly in connection with teaching hospitals. But, on the whole, most lunatics continued to be sent directly to rural asylums.[25]

The family-care system was an alternative care program designed for the purpose of relieving overcrowded asylums. In 1883 Massachusetts undertook a program of boarding out lunatics who were quiet "and not dangerous nor committed as a dipsomaniac or inebriate."[26] In twenty years, of 762 lunatics who were boarded out with 462 families, there were only two suicides and no homicides. In 1907 Owen Copp, executive officer, Massachusetts State Board of Insanity, reported that the experiment had been eminently successful. Yet, he stated, "The potentiality of danger is inherent, as in all other dealings with the insane, who are unstable and may veil vicious motives and tendencies in apparently harmless guises."[27]

Only a few of the younger medical superintendents followed the example of trial discharges and boarding-out. Most alienists believed that the safest course was to commit all the insane and to discharge reluctantly. But, at the theoretical level, practitioners continued to identify only specific types of mental disorder with dangerousness, but they believed that all lunatics were liable to "paroxysms."

# Homicidal Insanity and the Unstable Nervous System 1870–1910

6

The change to a strictly neurophysiological view of insanity fostered the theoretical modification of several diagnostic concepts. Rudolf Virchow's cell theory supported the concept of inflammation and renewed interest in the role that the circulation of blood, by now at the capillary level, played in producing mental symptoms. Alienists reevaluated the static states of partial insanity in this new light. The existence of such pathological events as moral insanity and monomania were rejected outright by some physicians and reinterpreted by others.[1]

## Intellectual Insanity: Dementia Praecox and Paranoia

During the 1880s, the concept of monomania or homicidal insanity underwent theoretical change, but the belief that the lunatic laboring under delusions and command hallucinations was dangerous prevailed. Because the idea of partial insanity, that a person could be insane on one point and sane on all others, had been challenged by Gray, Bucknill and Tuke, Maudsley, and others, the finding of delusions in the course of a mental examination came to be diagnostic of far-reaching brain disorder. Some physicians continued to place the delusion in a position of diagnostic primacy, but others, conceding its global significance, maintained

**74**

nevertheless that insanity of an equally serious nature could occur without delusions. But it was generally agreed that the use of the term monomania to designate all sorts of morbid symptoms would result in the indefinite multiplication of monomanias, far removed from the original conception.[2]

By 1884 the term monomania was falling into disuse and was being replaced by a new idea. Although the term paranoia had been used in many ways since Hippocrates, its application to persecutory delusions originated in the psychiatric textbook of Richard Krafft-Ebing. The Germans used the term *Primäre Verrucktheit*. The essential characteristic of paranoia was delusions of persecution arising out of an antecedent emotional disturbance, yet not progressing to dementia.[3] Although the nomenclature changed, the relationship between delusions and homicidal insanity remained constant in the minds of physicians.[4]

### The Freeman Case

In certain states, the lunatic who committed homicide was designated as permanently dangerous. Under some of these laws, no provision was made for discharge from the asylum after recovery. For example, in Massachusetts in 1879 Charles F. Freeman murdered his child under the delusion that the Lord had commanded the sacrifice. The governor sent him directly to the Danvers Lunatic Hospital without trial. By 1883 Freeman had recovered and was brought before the supreme court for a sanity hearing. The alienists gave no conflicting testimony in describing his recovery from the delusion. The result was that he was declared "not guilty by reason of insanity." Under the 1873 Massachusetts law, "when a person is acquitted of murder or manslaughter on the ground of insanity he must, regardless of his condition at the time of his acquittal, be committed to one of the lunatic hospitals for life." Alienist Charles F. Folsom, who reported the case, interpreted the spirit of the law as punitive rather than for the protection of the public: "Has any sane man escaped punishment by the Massachusetts law, so far as is known?"[5]

## The Webber Case

Public opinion overrode psychiatric theory in some cases, even when the existence of delusions and their direct connection with the homicide was unequivocal. Since the Guiteau trial, public sentiment favored executing offenders who were not flagrantly deranged.[6] The neurologist William A. Hammond lent substantial support to this position. Since 1873 he had publicly advocated executing the homicidal insane both as an example to other lunatics and to protect the public.[7]

The Webber murder case in Philadelphia in 1887 illustrates the way in which lay sentiment overpowered expert testimony. Testimony by physicians and by Webber's family and friends established the history of a previously sane man, free of criminal influences and associations, who in the autumn of 1885 began to show a change of character as well as disposition and the growing presence of irrational beliefs. He was convinced that his wife chloroformed him and received visits from her lovers. He believed that he was pursued and persecuted by members of his family, friends, and fellow workmen. On December 6, 1886, he shot and killed William H. Martin, a jeweler, in his shop. No motive or connection between the two men could be found.[8]

The only witnesses called to rebut the testimony of Webber's intimates and the alienists were the police officer who arrested him, the magistrate who committed him, the turnkey, the police lieutenant of the district, and the coroner who held the inquest. All testified to the man's calmness and self-possession, which they believed to be evidence of sanity. The commonwealth argued to the jury that it was a case of simulated insanity "on the part of a vicious and bad tempered man." The jury returned the verdict of murder in the first degree.

Every effort was made from a legal standpoint to obtain a new trial. On March 19, 1888, the state supreme court affirmed the judgment of the lower court, and Webber was subsequently executed. One question that remained unanswered about the case was why he was not committed as a dangerous lunatic before the homicide took place. In September 1886 his wife went to live with her father on the advice of the family physician. Evidently both recognized the dangerousness in Webber, but he was not committed, a relatively simple procedure in Pennsylvania at that time.

### Emotional Insanity: Moral Insanity and Homicidal Impulse

The idea of a mental disorder that was confined to the emotions remained the subject of intense controversy. Some physicians continued to believe that unless lunatics were delusional or demented, they were sane and responsible. These doctors rejected the existence of mental disorders characterized by morbid emotions or uncontrollable impulses. They did not deny that humans suffered from such states of mind, but they believed that such conditions were moral problems, not insanity. As Carlson and Dain have pointed out, psychiatric writers continued as before to discuss rigorously the conditions in which dangerousness was motivated by morbid emotions, and they continued to defend their theoretical position in Association meetings and other professional forums.[9]

An example of this kind of discussion occurred at the 1872 meeting of the Association when, after having heard John Curwen, superintendent of the Pennsylvania State Lunatic Asylum, read a paper on "Diagnosis and Treatment of Insanity," William H. Compton, of the Lunatic Asylum at Jackson, Mississippi, rose to say: "I would like, however, to ask just one broad question . . . do we recognize moral insanity or not?" Kirkbride answered that some medical superintendents did and some did not, noting the difference of opinion between Ray and the *American Journal of Insanity*, namely, Gray. But again, as before another desultory discussion on moral insanity ensued without any resolution of the problem. Opponents continued to condemn the concept as mere rationalization of human depravity, the failure to overcome the effects of original sin. Gray remained adamant on the issue, as did Ordronaux. The editors of the *American Journal of Insanity* seized upon cases both from America and from abroad to discredit the idea of a purely emotional insanity.[10]

In addition to the medical superintendents who advocated the concept of moral insanity, the new force in the field, the neurologists, tended to accept the concept, drawing upon their neuro-physiological and hereditarian beliefs. The editorial position of the *Journal of Nervous and Mental Disease* in 1877 was that it was *a priori* impossible for a discrete moral faculty to exist. Some advocates believed that the somatic theory of insanity in fact favored the existence of the moral faculty as separate from the intellectual.[11]

### Weakened or Absent Moral "Sense"

Despite disagreements about the theoretical possibility of moral insanity, physicians continued to report this type of case in the literature. By the turn of the century, owing in part to the influence of the degeneracy theory, the concept of a moral imbecility became more prominent. This term referred not only to the feebleminded, the idiot, and the imbecile, but to persons who had normal intellectual powers in which the moral principle was absent.[12] In 1883, for example, the neurologist Edward Spitzka stated: "There are subjects whose reasoning powers are fair, whose memory is excellent, who are perhaps, accomplished in the arts, but in whom the moral sense is either deficient or entirely absent. The term *moral insanity* of authors should be limited to this class of subjects, and a much better term to use would, in the writer's opinion, be MORAL IMBECILITY."[13]

### The Case of William B.

Some alienists held that the absence or weakening of the moral sense made the lunatic dangerous. C. K. Clarke, of the Rockwood Hospital, Kingston, Ontario, reported an example of moral imbecility. The lunatic, William B., had a childhood history of torturing and killing birds as well as raping little girls. In 1870 he was committed to Rockwood Criminal Asylum for raping a child, the death sentence having been commuted to life imprisonment. In 1878 he was pardoned for good conduct and set free. He promptly stole a horse and mutilated it; when this was dis-

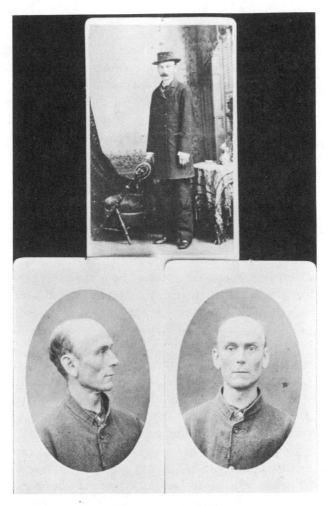

William B. Moral imbecility referred to those in whom the moral principle was weakened or absent—not only to the feebleminded, but also to persons with normal intelligence. Medical Superintendent C. K. Clarke wrote of William B.: "No one could see him so engaged [in reading the newspapers, conversing, and playing cards] and believe that he was naturally so vicious and depraved." C. K. Clarke, "The Case of William B.: Moral Imbecility," *American Journal of Insanity*, 43 (1886). (Courtesy, The Ohio State University Health Sciences Library)

covered, the authorities captured him once again and committed him to jail as a dangerous lunatic.[14]

William B. was then admitted to the Rockwood Asylum, where he persistently tortured fellow patients. He was able to accumulate all kinds of sharp objects, such as forks, nails, and pins, and delighted in sticking pins into the flesh of old and feeble patients. On one occasion, he hid a helpless one under a rubbish pile in the basement of the asylum, intending to return later to torture him, but the attendants discovered the plan before he was able to carry it through.

On August 20, 1884, William B. eloped during an outing and was recaptured while in the act of raping a little girl. He was then sent to jail for six months. The jailer did not believe he was insane and gave him a job as a cook. Dr. Davison, of the asylum, sent a letter to the supervisor of the jail, warning of B.'s dangerousness; the authorities, however, were still not convinced he was insane. Indeed, Clarke reported that he was intelligent and literate: "No one could see him so engaged [in reading the newspapers, conversing, and playing cards] and believe he was naturally so vicious and depraved."[15]

By the end of the century, alienists accepted the accumulated clinical observations, and the controversy surrounding the moral imbecility concept weakened. Emil Kraepelin, whose first edition of the *Textbook* appeared in 1883, placed the concept squarely within the context of the degeneracy theory. Moral imbecility became a harbinger of continuous degeneration of all faculties. In 1904 the alienist Henry R. Stedman reported the case of J. T., a professional nurse who fatally poisoned twenty people. Stedman was one of three medico-legal experts called to examine the prisoner. On the basis of her social and family history, the nature of her crimes, and her mental status during the investigation, Stedman and his colleagues concluded that "the prisoner's disease history and present mental state correspond with a well-recognized form of mental defect of a moral type due to congenital degeneration, in which there may be little or no intellectual disturbance that is apparent to the ordinary observer." On June 3, 1902, J. T. was tried and found not guilty by reason of insanity and committed to a state hospital for life. Stedman followed the case at the Taunton Massachusetts Insane Hospital and documented her continued mental degeneration. During the second year of her confinement there, she developed delusions that the food was poisoned, thus supporting Stedman's contention that "intellectual involvement in some form, is an essential feature of the disease . . . that there is no such thing as a mental disorder affecting the moral sphere alone." The constitutional nature of the disease made recovery impossible, and "if ever at large again she would be a constant menace to the community."[16]

In 1908 William Alanson White, of the Government Hospital for the Insane, in a widely used textbook, described the "psychopathic constitution." He postulated that, though this set of behaviors did not properly constitute insanity, the difficulties of adjustment with the environment experienced by such individuals often made them insane. Among these various constitutional anomalies were those cases of pronounced defects in character that were seen in the criminal classes. White classified these cases as moral imbeciles.[17] With the rise of dynamic psychiatry in the second decade of the twentieth century, the psychiatric symptoms of these lunatics would be of increasing interest and significance.

### Homicidal Impulse

The concept of homicidal impulse, or homicidal monomania, underwent theoretical change toward the end of the century, but the clinical phenomenon continued to be reported in the literature. The essential clinical features were: (1) an intrusive idea to commit homicide; and (2) full awareness by the lunatic of its moral consequences. Some physicians, notably Gray and Ordronaux, rejected this phenomenon as a mental disorder, though, again, they did not deny the existence of such a human experience.[18]

A significant number of physicians recognized the homicidal impulse as a form of dangerous insanity. The use of the term monomania in connection with this phenomenon was also being questioned as it was similarly challenged in connection with delusions. Spitzka was dissatisfied with the term: "Such persons have

THE AMERICAN JOURNAL OF INSANITY, Vol. LXI, No. 2.          PLATE XXVI.

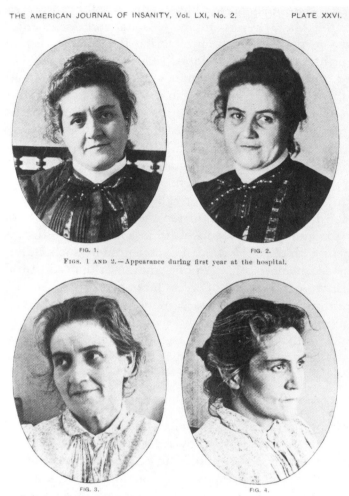

FIG. 1.                                    FIG. 2.

FIGS. 1 AND 2.—Appearance during first year at the hospital.

FIG. 3.                                    FIG. 4.

FIGS. 3 AND 4.—Appearance during second year at the hospital, after a period of refusal of food due to delusions of poisoning.

J. T., a professional nurse who fatally poisoned twenty people. Medico-legal experts involved in the case concluded that "the prisoner's disease history and present mental state correspond with a well-recognized form of mental defect of a moral type due to congenital degeneration." Henry R. Stedman, "A Case of Moral Insanity with Repeated Homicides and Incendiarism and Late Development of Delusions," *American Journal of Insanity*, 61 (1904). (Courtesy, The Ohio State University Health Sciences Library) been styled homicidal monomaniacs, . . . [but] patients with this symptom should be designated: lunatics with *insane homicidal impulses.*"[19] Others agreed that the homicidal impulse was symptomatic of a general derangement of the brain and was also an early sign of degeneration.[20]

## Cases of Neurasthenia

The principal clinicians accepted the existence of homicidal impulse as a symptom of a weakened condition of the nervous system. Contrary to the prominent belief that such morbid ideas and impulses were dangerous manifestations of hereditary degeneration, the neurologist Morton Prince reported a case in which he explained the homicidal impulse as a symptom of neurasthenia. The patient had acquired a neurasthenic condition after she was required to hold her sister while she was being etherized for a difficult birth. Thereafter, the patient, who was obliged to care for the child, was affected with the impulse to kill it. Prince reported, "Her psychosis consists, or has consisted for she is much better at present, of an *overwhelming fear* that she would kill the child, and an *impulse* to do this. . . . The fear and the impulse are not continuous, but come on paroxysmally without warning, at unexpected moments."[21] In all instances, the patient was able to resist the impulse to kill the baby, and Prince did not believe that she was dangerous. He never recommended restraint.

## Cases of "Pure Homicidal Impulse"

Alienists reported cases in which lunatics were unable to resist an imperative idea, as the phenomenon came to be called in the literature, to commit homicide. These cases kept alive the belief that such impulses were predictors of dangerousness. The British medical superintendent J. Wigglesworth in 1901 reported on a patient who, during her convalescence in the asylum, was seized with the desire to kill and nearly decapitated a fellow patient. The two had been assigned to work as domestics in the doctor's residence. On the morning of the incident, while at breakfast, he heard

desperate screaming from the third floor. There he found the patient in the process of severing the head of another convalescent
female. On the morning of the homicide, the former reported to
an attendant that she felt " 'desperate,' and experienced an uncontrollable desire to kill someone."[22] Evidently the attendant did
not take these feelings seriously or did not consider them to be
predictors of dangerousness.

### Homicidal Impulse As a Symptom

By the end of the nineteenth century, homicidal impulse, and impulses in general, came to be regarded as symptoms of psychiatric
illness, but not mental disease *sui generis*. After Kraepelin's clinical
description and classification of mental disorders appeared in the
United States, according to Menninger such impulses came to be
associated with the complicated symptomatology of dementia
praecox.[23] For example, in 1906 Charles W. Hitchcock, an alienist
in Detroit, Michigan, reported the case of a young man who awoke
one morning feeling physically ill, and, though during the course
of the ensuing hours he exhibited certain peculiarities of conduct,
he was not regarded as dangerous and therefore was not taken into
custody. He continued to be somewhat mentally confused and for
no reason he could recall boarded a train and travelled to the home
of his godmother, whom he murdered. His conduct during the day
prior to the homicide characterized his mental status as definitely
abnormal. Hitchcock concluded that "the purposeless impulsive
act . . . and vague and poorly systematized ideas of persecution"
were clearly symptoms of dementia praecox.[24]

As a symptom instead of a disease, the homicidal impulse became identified with two distinct mental conditions. In constitutional psychopathic states, a name given to the conditions
brought about by a degenerating nervous system, the homicidal
impulse, and impulses in general, were believed to be stigmata
of degeneracy. In dementia praecox, alienists saw the homicidal
impulse as evidence of the emotional indifference, deterioration
of the will, and the impulsive as well as purposeless behaviors
that were often destructive and dangerous. In the case of dementia

praecox, the patient did not seek help from an alienist or pray to be restrained by family and friends as did some patients with imperative ideas. Although some clinicians began to take note that such individuals did not always act upon these thoughts, sensational cases in the literature inclined practitioners to a continuing belief in the potential dangerousness of the homicidal impulse. By 1900 this impulse, therefore, inevitably signaled to physicians the presence of dementia praecox.

### Volitional Insanity: Mania Transitoria and Epilepsy

The existence of *mania transitoria* continued to be one of the most intensely debated issues of this period. The reality of a form of insanity that could arise instantaneously, run a short but intense course, and terminate in complete cure was diametrically opposed to a conception of insanity as physical disease. It has been noted that by 1860 alienists believed that *mania transitoria* was a phenomenon associated with epilepsy.

Some physicians reasoned that, on the basis of neurophysiology, a transitory condition was possible. Ray argued in favor of *mania transitoria* in 1871.[25] Spitzka in 1883 described "transitory frenzy," an identifiable condition "*of impaired consciousness, characterized by either an intense maniacal fury or confused hallucinatory delirium, whose duration does not exceed the period of a day or thereabouts.*"[26] Spitzka noted that some thinkers associated the phenomenon exclusively with epilepsy, but he said also that it would be a remarkable form of the disease that was limited to one attack in a lifetime and when other somatic manifestations of the disease were absent. He conceded that he had never seen a case of *mania transitoria*, but he accepted its existence on theoretical principle and on the reports of various authorities.[27]

Other physicians expressed reservations about the condition in the absolute absence of any known brain pathology. Maudsley, in 1874, maintained his position that the condition was associated with cerebral seizures that did not progress to *grand mal*. He stated, "Many cases of so-called transitory mania (*mania transitoria*) are really cases of this kind—cases of mental epilepsy."[28] Yet, he conceded that not all cases of *mania transitoria* were so explained. Because of the structure of the nervous system, it was within the boundaries of theoretical possibility, and Maudsley like Spitzka did not reject the existence of the disorder absolutely.[29]

A few physicians rejected the reality of *mania transitoria*. Ordronaux, for example, saw the disorder as a natural corollary to the false doctrine of moral insanity. He reasoned that all diseases show some relations to past and present physical states, but in *mania transitoria* nature changed all the rules. Gray also argued against the phenomenon on the same scientific grounds. He acknowledged that states of unpredictable paroxysmal mania were a common occurrence in pre-existing brain disease, but that the classic definition of *mania transitoria* could be applied to any case of crime that might be mentioned.[30] His position on this issue did not change from his original opinion in the Wright case in 1864.

### Mania Transitoria As "Temporary Insanity"

The temporary insanity of *mania transitoria* continued to be raised as a defense for homicide. In 1878 Carlos F. MacDonald, superintendent of the New York State Lunatic Asylum for Insane Criminals at Auburn, reported the case of Edmund J. Hoppin, who murdered the man who had abandoned Hoppin's sister after she had become pregnant. As a result of this adversity, the sister attempted suicide and the mother died. When the man returned to taunt the family, Hoppin seized a baseball bat and struck him on the head. Hoppin's attorney raised the plea of *mania transitoria*. Three alienists testified against the existence of the disorder, but the jury nonetheless voted for acquittal. MacDonald believed this occurred because of the shocking details of the story and the reputation of the Hoppin family, not because the jury believed that the defendant was in a state of temporary insanity. MacDonald concluded: "The time has arrived when it becomes the duty of the medical profession to set its face in opposition to the further progress of these chimerical, fallacious dogmas of 'transitory mania,' and 'homicidal impulse,' and to make some effort to eradicate from the public mind the false ideas which now pertain respecting the manifestations of mental disease."[31]

Support for the existence of *mania transitoria* as a distinct psychiatric disorder continued to come from neurophysiological theory. The link between cerebral circulation and mental disorder was a theme in French pathological anatomy for the first half of the nineteenth century. *Mania transitoria* could be explained in terms of a sudden increase in the blood supply to cerebral tissue. In Tuke's *Dictionary of Psychological Medicine* (1892), the contributor of the article on *mania transitoria* wrote: "We certainly believe that, as a rule, the typical *mania transitoria is produced by hyperaemia of the cortex of the brain.*" The causes of this hyperaemia were to be found in the cooperation of the many factors that could modify the blood supply to the brain, among others, "*strong drinks, mental excitement, physical and mental overwork, rapid change of temperature, indigestion and gastric disorders,* and *poisoning with carbon monoxide.*" Other factors or circumstances that could possibly produce the condition were sleep-drunkenness, and somnambulism.[32]

## The McFarland Case

The trial of Daniel McFarland in 1870 illustrates the extent to which the neurophysiological theory of *mania transitoria* could be carried to support the insanity defense. In 1857 he married his wife under false pretenses, claiming to be a lawyer with a burgeoning practice and a fine home in the West. After the ceremony, the truth emerged that he was a resident of a New York City lodging house who was given to heavy drinking. He had brutally abused his wife and their children.[33]

In 1866 Mrs. McFarland became acquainted with a Mrs. Calhoun, "who whispered in her ear the new gospel of 'women's rights.' "[34] Having become acquainted with another gentleman in the meantime, Mrs. McFarland put into practice the theories of her friend Mrs. Calhoun, namely, the right of a woman to get rid of a drunken, abusive husband. After the divorce, McFarland shot his ex-wife's paramour when he learned that she intended to re-marry.

McFarland was tried for murder and the insanity defense was used. Three New York neurologists testified in support of the diagnosis of *mania transitoria*. R. A. Vance, R. L. Parsons, and W. A. Hammond all testified that McFarland's symptoms were indicative of congestion of the brain, and that the ophthalmoscope was employed to diagnose it. Hammond testified that he had used that instrument to ascertain the presence of congestion and the dynamograph to measure the strength of the nerves. He showed McFarland photographs of his ex-wife and spoke of her relationship with the victim, and "when the poor man [was] almost frantic with grief, . . . [he] found the pulse to be 142. At this time McFarland was almost uncontrollable, and exhibited all the symptoms of acute mania."[35] On the basis of this expert testimony, McFarland was acquitted.

The case generated considerable public and professional outrage. Gray was outspoken in the matter and had reprinted in the *American Journal of Insanity* the entire article on the subject from the British *Journal of Mental Science*. Both Gray and Thomas S. Clouston, editor of the British journal, acknowledged the existence of transient states of violent mania, but only as an event within an already established mental disease. They attacked the absurdity of both the content and the method of the examination of McFarland as well as Hammond's touting of unsubstantiated theory as medical fact.

The essential nature of *mania transitoria* rendered the phenomenon absolutely unpredictable. Even the presence of hereditary taint was equivocal. The etiological factors and the circumstances were so widely varied that there was no way of predicting the manner in which any of these variables would come together to precipitate the condition. Further, the most reliable predictor, a previous occurrence, did not apply in this case because alienists believed that *mania transitoria* occurred only once in a person's lifetime.[36]

By the 1890s, belief in an idiopathic *mania transitoria* had dissolved, and, though some theorists did not disbelieve outright the old reports in the literature, physicians tended to reinterpret these cases in terms of an underlying neuropathology, such as alcohol ingestion, parturition, and, most often, epilepsy.[37] During the last decade of the century, the concept of a purely idiopathic *mania transitoria* faded away.

### Epileptic Insanity

By 1870, because of the belief in hereditary degeneracy and the neurophysiological bases for insanity, physicians conceived of epilepsy as a more formidable condition than they had in the 'fifties and 'sixties. The phenomenon of epileptic insanity was well described in the literature. The epileptic came to be regarded as unpredictable and dangerous, even in the absence of seizures.

Neurophysiological research cast light upon the nature of the epileptic seizure and the psychic phenomena associated with the paroxysms. John Hughlings Jackson was the most instrumental in epilepsy research. He posited the idea that the mental disorders, from slight confusion to homicidal mania, were a result of dissolution of the nervous system, a principle that he had taken from Herbert Spencer. The highest coordinating centers of the cerebrum, meaning those acquired most recently in the process of evolution, were affected first in a seizure; voluntary control was lost and automatisma remained. In Jackson's opinion, this principle applied not only to epilepsy, but to insanity in general.[38]

Not all homicides by epileptics were excused. As in other partial insanities, alienists and neurologists did not agree among themselves about the diagnosis of this condition or about the legal culpability of the epileptic. Conflicting testimony sent a number of such individuals to the gallows.[39]

### Epilepsy and Insane Homicide

Alienists and neurologists identified three clinical states that made the epileptic dangerous. First, the state of consciousness that preceded or followed a seizure made the patient potentially capable of grisly crime that was described in the literature in the most histrionic terms.[40] Epileptic furor or mania could be associated with both the *petit mal* or *grand mal* seizure. Ordronaux reported such a case in 1875. Isabella Jenisch, after a *grand mal* seizure, put her four-year-old daughter into the stove, burning the lower half of the child's body. The girl survived for thirty-six hours, during which the mother seemed insensible and stuporous, disinterested in the child's suffering.[41]

Second, the phenomenon of masked epilepsy (*epilepsie larvée*), described by Esquirol, Morel, Burrows, and others, occurred when the seizure did not progress to a *grand mal* but was manifested in unconscious, automatic behavior, often of the most violent and destructive character. Although some doubt arose about whether masked epilepsy was a unique phenomenon rather than a post-epileptic state, physicians accepted its existence into the twentieth century. A few alienists and neurologists, including Tuke, expressed doubt.[42] Other British and American alienists acknowledged masked epilepsy as a separate clinical phenomenon.[43]

Thirdly, the epileptic was dangerous because of the interparoxysmal mental state, or what physicians referred to as the "epileptic personality." The epileptic was described to be at all times quarrelsome, petty, easily offended, and unpredictably combative. Neurologists explained this personality in terms of moral generation or the epileptic's inability to control his animal instincts.[44]

Some alienists and neurologists maintained that the epileptic was essentially wicked. The popularized degeneracy theory and the religious belief in human depravity levied public and professional prejudice upon this "unfortunate class." Alienists and neurologists reasoned that epileptic automatisms took certain forms, such as public incontinence, undressing, profanity, and the like because of the epileptic's depravity.[45] Manuel Echeverria, an alienist who wrote extensively on epilepsy, believed that "we are never safe with them."[46]

## Asylums for Epileptics

Alienists and lay people alike agitated for the institutionalization of all epileptics. By the end of the century, only two state legislatures had funded such asylums. The Ohio Hospital for Epileptics received its first patients in 1893, and New York's Craig Colony for Epileptics followed the next year. The asylums protected the public from the epileptic and vice versa.[47] The medical superintendents of both these institutions expressed their belief publicly that epileptics were liable to attack others frequently with deadly violence.[48]

These patients were neither sedated, restrained, nor closely supervised. Except for the acutely ill and demented, all others lived in cottages housing twenty-five to a hundred residents. Physicians assigned individuals to the various cottages according to their skills and physical abilities. As in all state institutions of the period, the inmates made a substantial contribution to the material management of the physical plant.

The concentration of large numbers of epileptics did not precipitate the anticipated violence. From November 1893 to November 1909 some 4,281 epileptics had been admitted to the Ohio Hospital; yet, the medical superintendents reported only one death caused by the attack of another epileptic. Despite an annual increase in the census and many additions to the physical plant, year after year medical superintendents of both institutions reported casualties that resulted from injuries sustained during violent convulsions or accidents that occurred while the patient was confused or unconscious following a convulsion. Neither the epileptic personality nor epileptic automatisms was the source of any fatal casualties.

Despite this evidence to the contrary, medical superintendent William H. Pritchard of the Ohio Hospital nevertheless held to his belief in the dangerousness of the epileptic. In his annual report of 1909, he asserted that the epileptic was "dangerous to others. During the mental disturbance which precedes, replaces or follows an attack he frequently commits acts of violence or may be guilty of homicide or other revolting crimes for which he is not really responsible."[49] William D. Spratling, the first medical superintendent of the Craig Colony for Epileptics, also believed that the affliction was characterized by the "meanest violence."[50] Yet Craig Colony was as free from injuries as the Ohio Hospital.

Belief in the epileptic personality and the dangerousness of epileptics persisted well into the twentieth century. So long as no effective anticonvulsant drug was available, many epileptics had no choice but to remain in these colonies or in state hospitals. Alienists forged a theoretical link between the violence of the *grand mal* seizure and the potential for dangerousness in these patients that would not weaken until the first specific anticonvulsant drug was introduced in 1938.

### The Phenomenology of Homicidal Insanity

By the last decades of the century, alienists had accumulated substantial clinical data about homicidal insanity. Some physicians believed that only the delusional or the unconscious were dangerous at the one extreme, and other specialists believed that any family history of insanity or epilepsy made the person dangerous. Most doctors rejected both extremes and tended to believe that dangerousness could arise from psychiatric disorders characterized by delusions and command hallucinations, lack of moral restraint, homicidal impulses, and the mania, or frenzy of epilepsy, though the names of the disorders had changed.

John P. Gray was one thinker who maintained an extreme position on this issue. His role in medico-legal cases and his contributions to any discussion on these matters at Association meetings have been noted throughout this volume. In 1875 he published a compendium of all cases of attempted and completed insane homicides admitted since 1843 to the New York Lunatic Asylum—125 cases in all. He concluded: "Delusion is the motive, which in most cases controls the conduct of the insane," though only 94 cases were attributed to delusion.[51]

Another study, of the female criminal lunatics at Broadmoor Asylum, in London, in 1901, supported Gray's findings. John Baker, deputy superintendent of the asylum said: "The type of insanity most commonly observed amongst these lunatic criminals is delusional mania." Of these cases of criminal lunacy, 253 women had killed their children, and 33 had attempted to do so but were prevented, the largest single sample. Baker pointed out that homicidal and suicidal tendencies were present "in at least one third of the cases of puerperal insanity, but that, as a rule, they are neither vicious, nor deliberate, nor well-directed. Vicious, no; but deliberate and well-directed, yes."[52] Clearly, psychiatrists assigned the position of primacy of delusions as predictors of dangerousness.

The rise of dynamic psychiatry brought about momentous theoretical changes over the next half century. But, rather than being overshadowed by these developments, somatic psychiatry made significant advances concurrently. Psychiatrists accounted for homicidal insanity and predicted dangerousness from both dynamic and somatic starting points.

# Psychoanalysis and Medical Criminology

**7**

During the first half of the twentieth century, up until the mid-1960s, American psychiatry was deeply affected by theoretical changes and practical discoveries that altered clinical practice. By 1910 many of the old-guard asylum superintendents had passed on, and a new generation of physicians had arrived. These psychiatrists embraced the standards of German medicine that had already motivated the neurologists to express their disdain for the isolated asylum superintendents. Although clear boundaries existed between neurology and psychiatry, by 1910 all physicians of the mind generally agreed about the ideal standards of psychiatric medicine.

Despite a common ideal of scientific medicine, after 1910 psychiatry included two distinct theories. The somatic theory of insanity that had prevailed since the beginning of the specialty was given impetus by German positivist medicine and discoveries about the cause of general paralysis (tertiary syphilis of the brain) as well as pellagrous insanity. The influence of the Italian criminologist Cesare Lombroso, who postulated the existence of a criminal brain based upon anatomical and physiological pathology, was deeply felt.

During the first decade of the century, however, psychoanalytic psychiatry became a force in American medicine. One reason for the rapid growth of psychoanalytic thought was that it provided a new paradigm for conceiving mental illness where the somatic model had so far failed. It was true that, though a number of casual relationships between mental phenomena and organic brain disease were established during this period, psychiatry lacked a unified theory; mental events such as delusions or depression could be explained from either a somatic or a dynamic starting point. After 1910 the two ways of explaining mental illness in general and dangerousness in particular were intertwined.[1]

Historians have identified the theoretical and social movements as well as the events that characterized the growth and evolution of psychiatry throughout this period. Advances in theory and classification of mental disorders reflected a growing body of empirical knowledge and a change in what psychiatrists considered relevant empirical data. Further, the formulation of a psychodynamic model of mental illness affected all areas of theory and practice. Concurrent development of specific somatic therapies kept the somatic model alive. Finally, in the 1950s, the formulation of a specific antipsychotic drug revolutionized psychiatric care.[2]

The social context in which these changes occurred affected their meaning and evolution. Traditional research on the Progressive movement has shown that psychiatrists were among the enlightened elite, who believed in the stewardship of the elect. The mental hygiene movement, eugenics, medical criminology, and the growth of dynamic psychiatry were all dependent upon a fundamental belief in the environment as the source of human problems and the ability of man to modify it.[3]

Psychiatrists' response to the social and military tragedies of World War I enhanced the progress of psychiatric theory and the prestige of the specialty. The period from 1905 to 1918, the Progressive period in the United States, was characterized by the growth of American scientific psychiatry and an independence from British influence. From 1918 until the 1950s, no aspect of American psychiatry, theoretical or practical, was left uninvestigated or unchallenged.[4]

What is striking is that, despite all of this growth in medicine, science, the psychiatric profession, and society in general, neither the character of dangerous insanity nor the disposition of the dangerous mental patient changed to any degree. Not even the popular concerns about returned soldiers of either World War with mental disabilities affected the thinking of psychiatrists on the subject of dangerousness. Some forms of dangerous insanity were given new names and explained in different ways, but the patients and problems remained essentially the same as those first identified by Pinel, Rush, Esquirol, Prichard, Ray, and Conolly.

### Dynamic Psychiatry and Homicidal Insanity

The work of Sigmund Freud first came to the attention of American psychiatrists during the first decade of the century. The evolution of psychoanalytic psychiatry in this country has been chronicled by Oberndorf, Burnham, Hale, Quen and Carlson, Sicherman, and others. These historians agree that psychiatry's reception of psychoanalytic ideas was facilitated by George M. Beard's concept of neurasthenia and the thinking of S. Weir Mitchell and Morton Prince, all neurologists. In fact, the psychotherapy movement in the United States was initiated by neurologists.[5]

Another factor in the reception of psychoanalytic thought was the change in psychiatric assessment initiated by Adolf Meyer at the close of the nineteenth century. In 1896, while clinical director of the Worcester Asylum, he went to Heidelberg to study with Kraepelin and later introduced Kraepelinian diagnostic categories into American hospitals. As neuropathologist first at the Illinois State Hospital and then at the Worcester Asylum, he had conducted post-mortem examinations on hundreds of deceased patients. He was trained in the best tradition of German medicine and had studied under Jean Charcot in Paris and John Hughlings Jackson in England.

Meyer was brought to Worcester to improve the scientific work of the asylum. Yet he concluded that the mind could not be found in the brain but in the interaction of the whole biology of the person and his life history.[6] He introduced the study of the whole patient in terms of the life history and personality reactions in all areas of human existence: psychological, social, cultural, and organic. Whereas the clinical empiricists, exemplified by Kraepelin, sought only to describe the objective properties of the person as a clinical entity, Meyer sought in the intrapsychic life history as well as the adaptive habits of the patient the key to understanding the illness.

Although this approach to psychiatry was not considered "dynamic" in the strict sense, Menninger notes that Meyer's theories represented a departure from somatic psychiatry. Meyer believed that dementia praecox was a pathological response to environmental stress rather than a specific disease entity. In fact, at the famous 1909 Clark University celebration at which Freud spoke, he read a paper in which he postulated the dynamic factors in dementia praecox and elaborated his conception of the phenomenon as the outcome of inadequate reactions to the environment and habit deterioration.[7]

Under the influence of psychoanalysis (Freud) and "psychobiology" (Meyer) as well as other contemporary thinking, psychiatrists formulated new conceptualizations of homicidal insanity. Freud's theory of the homosexual origins of paranoia was widely discussed, for example.[8] In 1929 Gregory Zilboorg, of the New York Hospital, who trained in both Vienna and Berlin, postulated somewhat different explanations for psychosis related to parenting, especially death wishes against children.[9] In 1934 Lauretta Bender, of New York's Bellevue Hospital, suggested that child murder by parents was not an expression of conscious or unconscious hatred, but rather the projection of symptoms onto the child so that he or she became the hypochondriacal object. This type of murder may represent the generic suicidal drive.[10]

Another example of psychoanalytic explanation for dangerousness was related to epilepsy. In 1919 L. Pierce Clark read a paper before the American Psychopathological Association in which he postulated that epilepsy was "an outflow from a homosexual component which is not sublimated or accepted . . . epileptic makeup . . . being deep rooted in narcissism which results from poorly repressed homosexuality."[11] Clark suggested that, instead of the outward projections of the paranoiac, the epileptic attacked his own body. This view ultimately lost out to both somatic and other psychodynamic interpretations, but it, too, illustrates the urgent attempts of dynamic psychiatrists to search out the causes of dangerous behavior.

Freud remarked in an interview while at Clark University that the psychoanalytic cure was "best suited to severe cases," but, in fact, the major impact of dynamic psychiatry in this country was in the treatment of nonpsychotic patients in extra-asylum treatment settings. Quen suggests that dynamic psychiatry increased the burdens and inadequacies of the state hospital system and resulted to a certain extent in the abandonment of the hospitalized insane.[12]

## Decline of the State Hospitals

By 1890 mental institutions were changing their names from asylum to hospital and eliminating the words "lunatic" and "insane" from the terminology. Twenty-nine institutions in the United States and Canada had done so by 1894, reflecting cultural advances and the beginning of Progressivism rather than any noteworthy change in the medical treatment of the insane. It is true that by then psychiatry was imbued with the spirit of German empiricism, but, aside from increased pathological investigations, the medical care of the insane in institutions had not made any noticeable progress. Advances were limited to the elaboration of hydrotherapy and occupational therapy. The presence of uniformed nurses, mostly products of asylum training schools that were hastily established, reinforced the appearance of scientific medicine.[13]

During the first decade of the century, psychiatrists sought to refine and standardize the assessment process. Meyer devised a scheme for the assessment of the whole person's life history. William A. White, of the Government Hospital for the Insane, in Washington, formulated a standardized assessment, but neither his scheme nor Meyer's specified any special test for dangerousness. White advocated a combination of what is now the standard neurological assessment and mental-status examination, "mainly by the conversational method." Although directions for examination of the psychiatric patient had been included in the textbooks from abroad since the mid-nineteenth century, the process of assessment after the turn of the century placed more emphasis upon life histories and intrapsychic processes.[14]

Despite this flurry of medical activity and optimism during the Progressive period, asylums remained vastly overcrowded. The rise of outpatient clinics, psychiatric units in general hospitals, and office psychiatry undoubtedly kept some nonpsychotic patients out of institutions. Involuntary commitment and isolation in the locked ward, however, remained the standard disposition of homicidal patients. Special hospitals continued to be erected for the criminally insane in various states, but homicidal patients were still present in the wards of many state mental hospitals.

Although conditions in many of these institutions had been deteriorating since the late nineteenth century, during the economic depression of the 1930s most of them experienced a period of rapid and irreversible decline. Many were jammed and lacked personnel. In 1934 John Maurice Grimes, a member of the Council on Medical Education and Hospitals of the American Medical Association, published the results of a two-year study of all types of mental institutions. He reported that in many of them all available space had been requisitioned for sleeping quarters. Beds were brought in or pallets were made up on the floors of hallways, dining rooms, gymnasiums, amusement halls, between other beds, and in hydrotherapy rooms. Inadequate supervision made locked doors and barred windows a necessity. Patients could receive little or no medical attention because the average ratio of physicians to patients was only 1:228. Furthermore, the turnover of medical personnel was rapid because of low salaries and political influence. State hospitals employed few registered nurses, and some none at all. Grimes remarked, "patients are taken physically ill, remain so for days or perhaps weeks, and recover or die without the service of registered nurses."[15]

## Reluctance to Discharge

The nineteenth century reluctance to discharge recovered and improved patients continued into the twentieth century and was a major factor in the overcrowding problem. In view of the enormous number of patients and the ease of admission to mental hospitals, individual assessment did not likely go beyond the receiving wards and the diagnostic process. Kraepelin had observed that in dementia praecox, the diagnosis given most twentieth-century patients, the prognosis was unfavorable. Individuals therefore became trapped in locked wards for long periods of time—months sometimes extending into years—for they were classified from the outset as incurable.

When, during World War I, public mental hospitals experienced a major nationwide shortage of personnel, clinical directors began to establish schemes to release as many patients as possible. By this time, the role of the social worker was well established, and so most of these schemes involved transition care. Candidates for parole were selected with care; only those who had functioned well in work roles within the asylum were included. Known homicidal patients were, of course, excluded. The results of these experiments led researchers to conclude that more than half of the patients selected for parole were able to remain in the community.[16]

### Escapes from Mental Hospitals

Although the patients in the parole schemes were selected with care, some could and did leave hospitals against medical advice and a substantial number escaped. A study of escapes from the Chicago State Hospital from July 1, 1918, to June 30, 1919, showed that, of the 431 men involved, 308 were promptly returned to police, family, or friends. But 123 were never heard from again. A vigorous social service follow-up revealed the fate of only 25. Of this group, only 4 had made an "adequate adjustment," according to the psychiatrists, but no cases of assault or homicide were reported. The authors of the study concluded: "Certainly there is no justification for the terrifying picture so often painted by the press of the dangerous *moron* rushing madly from the asylum for the sole purpose of gratifying his perverted desires at the expense of the innocent and unprotected."[17]

Studies of patients discharged against medical advice from St. Elizabeth's Hospital from 1920 to 1926 and from the Boston Psychopathic Hospital in 1925 showed similar results. Of the 385 patients included in these studies, only 2 from the St. Elizabeth's group "committed major crimes," though their nature was not specified. No crimes were reported in the Boston group. The psychiatrists in both studies drew the conclusion that it was difficult for even the most skilled practitioner to predict dangerousness. These psychiatrists found their results both positive and surprising.[18]

Psychiatrists continued to believe that complete recovery from mental illness was unlikely and that mental patients were a menace, if not a positive danger, to the community. This belief contributed to the reluctance to discharge patients and the overcrowding that taxed the ability of the staff to offer individual care. Ironically, fatal accidents would probably have been avoided if the predictably dangerous patient could have been more closely watched.[19]

## The Rise of Medical Criminology

Another result of progressivism and psychoanalytic thought was the study of individual criminals. Central to medical criminology was the belief that the cause of this type of behavior was to be found in the internal conflicts of individuals and their reactions to his environment. During the first decade of the twentieth century, psychiatrists challenged the concepts of depravity and innate criminality.

These theories were articulated in publications beginning with William Healy's The Individual Delinquent in 1915. His thesis was that delinquency was environmentally determined. William A. White reiterated this theme in *Insanity and the Criminal Law*, which was published in 1923. He claimed that criminology "is dominated by a belief in psychological determinism . . . as well as in the purely physical, whatever takes place can be explained by what went before and out of which it developed."[20]

The evolution of dynamic psychiatry's approach to the criminal came to fruition in the case of Leopold and Loeb in 1924. Defense attorney Clarence Darrow used as witnesses dynamic psychiatrists, who retrospectively found explanations for the murderers' behavior in their life histories. These experts showed how non-intellectual factors could operate consistently in an individual's life.[21] The Leopold and Loeb case reaffirmed psychiatrists' belief that persons who were not appreciably defective in reason could be dangerous.

Psychiatric criminologists identified biological, dynamic, and environmental causes of dangerousness. They formulated schemes for examining offenders that spelled out special approaches and techniques which took into consideration individual temperament and mentality. Benjamin Karpman, of the Government Hospital for the Insane, for example, maintained that crime and insanity were reducible to a common genesis in psychogenic need. Most criminologists, however, tended to identify a variety of sources and motivations for deviant behavior, including mental illness.[22]

Psychiatrists recognized the existence of various degrees of responsibility, thus keeping the theoretical issue of partial insanity viable. Criminologists generally recognized that insane and mentally deficient persons could act from motives that they themselves knew were antisocial. The study of the individual criminal reinforced this belief and fostered debate between the psychiatric and the legal professions about the role of punishment for the partially insane. Implicit in this discussion, however, was the question of how dangerous this type of offender was and how such dangerousness could be predicted and prevented. The perennial question was not one of fact, but one of disposition.[23]

### The Homicidal Insane in Hospitals

Psychiatrists seeking to define the nature of homicidal insanity by studying inmates in the few hospitals for the criminally insane, attempted to identify the diagnostic categories in which criminality was the predominant feature. Although a strict faculty psychology was no longer the basis for Kraepelinian classification, the recognition that mental illness was characterized by disordered thinking, feeling, and willing was implicit in the way in which alienists described their patients.

In one typical study in 1917, Paul E. Bowers, medical superintendent of the Indiana Hospital for Insane Criminals, described the most predominant forms of "mental alienation which often leads to crime; these are epilepsy, paranoia and feeble-mindedness." Of the paranoiac, he remarked: "The most dangerous of all insane patients is the one who harbors in the recesses of his diseased mentality systematized delusions of persecution." But Bowers also believed that feeblemindedness was the most common cause of crime. In his study, homicide and assault were the least represented categories. More than half of the criminally insane patients included in the study had committed petit or grand larceny, and only 19.8 percent murder or manslaughter. Bowers believed, however, that every burglar was a potential murderer.[24]

In another study, of 646 patients admitted to the Matteawan State Hospital from October 1, 1912, to July 1, 1918, the data showed that homicides and assaults were committed by patients diagnosed with dementia praecox, alcoholic psychosis, constitutional inferiority, and mental deficiency. Although most of these offenses were attributable to patients diagnosed as suffering from dementia praecox (31 of 113), patients with alcoholic psychosis committed 25 of the total. However, 304 patients were incarcerated in Matteawan for the crimes of public intoxication, disorderly conduct, vagrancy, and prostitution. Again, the largest group of criminal insane who committed the crimes of disorderly conduct and the like were those with dementia praecox (82 of the 304) and with alcoholic psychosis (64 of the 304).[25]

Additional studies of populations of criminal insane showed that the vast majority were not homicidal. A study of five hospitals for the criminally insane, published in 1930, showed that, of 3,028 subjects, 916 were designated as homicidal. The largest diagnostic group was, again, those with dementia praecox; of the 514 patients in this group, 291 had committed murder and 223 had been institutionalized because they had threatened homicide. The second largest diagnostic group was the paranoiacs; 70 had committed homicide and 74 were "homicidal."[26] Further, psychiatrists still identified patients with psychopathic personality and impulse disorder among the insane criminal populations.[27]

Criminologists swept all the dangerous insane into a common theoretical construct. Criminals were criminals whether they were petty thieves or paranoiacs. It followed that both were equally dangerous and deserved a common disposition. Well-known studies showed that the vast majority of patients in hospitals for the criminally insane were committed because they had been found guilty of theft, vagrancy, disorderly conduct, and other deeds of like magnitude.

During the first half of the twentieth century, American psychiatrists and neurologists shared a common ideal standard of scientific medicine. Proponents of both somatic and psychoanalytic theory formulated some new explanations for dangerous insanity, but those suffering from this condition did not benefit much from these new ideas. Despite the explicit interest of the new specialists, the criminologists, the care of dangerous lunatics did not change except for building more special asylums to house them.

Psychiatrists, who were uncertain about even the patient who had demonstrated no criminal propensities, were reluctant to discharge any from psychiatric hospitals. One result was the continued overcrowding of facilities and the inadequacy of personnel to provide care. The few psychiatrists who established successful programs of furlough and discharge tended to distrust their own results.

One benefit of this new vision of psychiatric medicine was that practitioners paid more attention to diagnostic techniques. They refined the method of assessing intrapsychic experience as well as life history and attempted to correlate laboratory data with other clinical findings. Criminologists were interested in the dynamic issues in the lives of dangerous lunatics. Yet, despite these technical advances and new ways of naming and classifying mental illness, psychiatrists continued to identify the same mental phenomena with homicidal insanity.

# Somatic and Dynamic Dangerousness 1910–1960

# 8

By 1910 Kraepelin's classification dominated psychiatric thought. His influence upon the system adopted by the New York State Commission in Lunacy in 1909 is obvious, for example. Still, Freud and his followers introduced a new order of concepts based upon psychoanalytic thought that challenged Kraepelin's conceptual framework. Psychiatric nomenclature continued to change over the next fifty years as practitioners theorized and debated about the essential nature of mental disorder.[1]

The phenomena associated with homicidal insanity remained the same, even though the nomenclature changed. In studies of large populations of the criminally insane, psychiatrists identified insane homicide associated with aberrations of intellection, emotion, and volition. These studies still demonstrated that homicide was most often identified with the thought disorders of dementia praecox and paranoia.[2] A substantial number of insane homicides were also attributed to conditions that, however named, were characterized by a lack of moral feelings or emotions, by psychopathic personality, and by mental deficiency. Finally, these tallies showed that patients with conditions characterized by a failure of behavior control, particularly epilepsy, committed insane homicide.

### Intellectual Insanity: Thought Disorder in Dementia Praecox

Anglo-American medical writers of the 'teens and 'twenties believed that insane homicide was positively associated with the peculiar disordered thought processes of dementia praecox. As psychiatrist Aaron J. Rosanoff, for example, stated in the sixth edition of his *Manual of Psychiatry* (1927): "It is not rare to encounter, especially in the beginning of the disease, attacks of very pronounced anxiety, suicidal ideas and attempts, or violent tendencies."[3] Frederick Peterson, in the ninth edition of *Nervous and Mental Diseases* (1919), associated delusions of persecution with insane homicide.[4]

In addition to, or subsequent to, disordered thought processes, psychiatrists regarded impulsive behavior patterns as dangerous and unpredictable. William A. White, in describing the symptoms of catatonic dementia praecox, wrote: "Quite characteristic of this condition, too are the *impulsive acts* of these patients. They will suddenly and with absolutely no warning whatever commit some act of violence. . . . The attacks come out of the clear sky, cannot be foreseen, and make these patients at times very dangerous."[5] Peterson, too, called attention to the dangerousness of impulsive behavior.[6]

Criminologists maintained that it was the characteristic impulsive behavior of patients with dementia praecox that largely accounted for their criminal tendencies. Criminologist Sheldon Glueck suggested in 1925 that these individuals were more the criminal type "than Lombroso's atavistic or epileptic, 'born criminal.' "[7] William Healy, in 1913 the director of the Juvenile Psychopathic Institute, in Chicago, related this example in his chapter on criminology that he contributed to White and Smith Ely Jelliffe's textbook:

. . . under the influence of morbid impulses and hallucinations, appearing early in the course of chronic mental disease, offenses may be committed, the psychopathological basis of which it may then be difficult to legally or even medically determine. A patient, after her marriage . . . became with her young husband greatly interested in religion, and they occupied themselves much with their devotions. During this access of piety, at one of her menstrual times, she heard the voice of God commanding her to raise her beloved mate out of this wicked world. She attempted homicidal assault, which was easily thwarted. Soon afterward, at another monthly period, she procured his revolver and shot him. He lived, but carried the bullet at the base of his skull. Then she was placed under observation in a private sanitarium where it is said that absolutely nothing out of the ordinary was observed. Her husband stated that it was then advised she become pregnant. A few months after giving birth to a child her menses reappeared, and with them the call came to get her child away from worldly contamination. She therefore battered in the side of its head against the table. Seen then in the hospital for several months she was quiet and well behaved. . . . Lacking the diagnosis of insanity . . . her treatment under the law could not consist of permanent detention against the wish of relatives, and once more she was taken out by them, became pregnant again, and . . . a few months after its birth, she effectually saved her second child from all earthly evils by putting it into the fire.[8]

Healy did not speculate about the dynamics of this patient's criminal behavior.

## Schizophrenia and Insane Homicide

Eugen Bleuler introduced the concept of schizophrenia as a dynamic interpretation of dementia praecox. But, up until 1924, when A. A. Brill translated Bleuler's textbook, Kraepelin's terminology still dominated the literature. Nevertheless, the concept gradually changed from a static to a dynamic interpretation. For example, in 1913 C. McFie Campbell, of Cornell Medical College and the Bloomingdale Asylum, suggested that Kraepelin ignored the dynamic relevance of psychotic symptoms, such as delusions, hallucinations, and impulsive behavior.[9]

Yet, the certain connection between schizophrenia and dangerousness soon became less apparent in the widely used textbooks. By the mid-1930s, neither Edward A. Strecker nor Arthur P. Noyes, both prominent dynamic psychiatrists, mentioned dangerousness or criminality in association with schizophrenia. Noyes, in 1934, discussed "impulsiveness and destructiveness" in connection with catatonic excitement. But broad statements about the unpredictability of schizophrenic patients were notably absent from Noyes's treatment of the subject. In fact, he never positively recommended involuntary commitment; he even expressed some reservations about asylum care in such cases.[10]

Strecker, like Noyes, focused upon the dynamics of the schizophrenic's thoughts, emotions, and behaviors rather than any dangerousness. In the second edition of the textbook written with Franklin G. Ebaugh, however, Strecker identified as a rare possibility dangerousness in connection with paranoid ideation. These authors reported a study of 200 consecutive cases of schizophrenia to show that paranoid ideas took widely variable forms and were not always evidence of dangerous insanity. Of these patients, the paranoid ideas in 34 were of the religious type; 31 had ideas of being drugged or poisoned; and 33 had poorly systematized delusions about Masons, Catholics, the Ku Klux Klan and the like. Only 20 of the 200 patients in the study, according to Strecker, were "actively homicidal."[11]

But psychiatrists maintained, however, that unintelligible or apparently motiveless crimes should *ex post facto* raise suspicions of schizophrenia. In 1948, Walter Bromberg stated: "The mechanisms which operate in the schizoid personality to cause aggressive crime unfortunately are not apparent until after the crime is committed." Bromberg suggested that schizophrenic patients sometimes committed homicide as a result of their self-destructive impulses being projected onto the victim: "Experience shows that apparently inexplicable brutal crimes which are perpetrated by psychopathic [mentally abnormal in the broad sense] individuals emerge from a matrix of emotional stress produced over a long period of conflict."[12]

Where the somatic psychiatrists tended to interpret the behavior of the psychotic patient in terms of hereditarian and physiological influences, the dynamic psychiatrists sought explanation for the behaviors, and the dangerous behavior in particular, within the context of the patient's life experiences. The dynamic interpretation, therefore, made homicidal insanity more difficult to predict.

One example of the failure to predict an insane homicide was the well publicized case of Bayard P. Peakes in 1953. He had been hospitalized on previous occasions and his psychiatrists were aware of his fixed delusion about the theoretical errors of modern physics. On the occasion of the homicide, he went to the Columbia University Physics Department to "kill some physicists" in order to draw attention to his opposition to J. Robert Oppenheimer's theories. But he arrived before any physicists, so he killed a secretary instead.[13]

Mid-century somatic and dynamic psychiatrists generally believed that the bizarre symptoms of schizophrenia were not in themselves predictors of dangerousness, but that command hallucinations, delusions, and impulsivity sometimes made these patients homicidal. But only rarely were the symptoms clear predictors of impending insane homicide. Both clinical psychiatrists and criminologists agreed that episodes of antisocial behavior, from petty crime to homicide, were signs of the insidious development of schizophrenia. Although the incipient schizophrenic could have committed a wide variety of petty crimes as a result of emotional detachment from his environment, the disordered thinking associated with the disease may also have led to impulsive or calculating behavior that would result in insane homicide.[14]

Practical advice on how to predict dangerousness in schizophrenic patients, even in discussions of paranoid schizophrenia, was notably absent from the standard textbooks after 1950. Psychiatrists theorized more about the dynamics of schizophrenia than the potential for insane homicide. Silvano Arieti, in the 1959 *American Handbook of Psychiatry*, stated only that escapes from the hospital and "homicidal impulses, at times successful, are more common in this group." Later psychiatrists tended to equivocate about whether or not patients who had delusions of persecution were dangerous. Where Arieti wrote in 1959 that homicidal impulses were "at times successful," Strecker had written of a case in 1925: "As this case indicates, the homicidal tendencies may be serious."[15]

## Paranoia

Psychiatrists after 1910 uniformly believed that the existence of paranoia as a pure disorder of the intellect was rare. They tended to conceive of it as the mental state in which fixed and systematized delusions of persecution were the chief clinical feature in terms of a continuum of paranoid states, which differed in a number of features from dementia praecox and other organic brain disorders, such as general paralysis (paresis), alcoholism, and senility.

Meyer, for example, contributing to White and Jelliffe's textbook in 1913, did recognize the implicit dangerousness of paranoia. Still, he maintained that psychiatrists, when treating patients, should not participate in their delusions. Although the ideal approach to the psychotherapy of paranoia was voluntary outpatient treatment, Meyer said, "It is not always easy to decide, when the patient's condition makes cooperation impossible and the right of protection of society becomes an absolute *duty*."[16] In the final analysis, Meyer conceded that the nature of the paranoid constitution required in most cases commitment to a closed institution.

Although psychiatrists differed widely in their beliefs about the etiology, treatment, and prognosis of paranoia (Peterson, for example, in 1919 believed that the prognosis was "absolutely unfavorable"), they agreed upon the point that delusions of persecution and reference made these patients dangerous.[17] Practitioners identified the typical forms; for example, *paranoia querulans* may lead to a lifelong involvement in the legal process and eventual attack upon the supposed tormentors. In *paranoia erotica*, danger could arise from the delusion that someone was interfering with the access of the lovers to one another. Peterson cited the case of one Dougherty, who followed the actress Mary Anderson all over the United States and threatened to kill anyone who interfered with his attempts to gain an interview. After he was committed to the asylum for these threats, he escaped but managed to return to murder one of the physicians.[18]

Identifiable stages in the development of paranoia were particularly meaningful to the dynamic psychiatrists. Meyer suggested that antisocial and dangerous acts could occur at any stage in the disease.[19] White, however, identified dangerousness specifically with the late second stage, when delusions of persecution and reference appeared. He wrote in 1919:

During this period of persecution the patient, when speaking of his persecutors, at first uses the pronoun "they." He is no more specific than this, but finally he may learn exactly who are at the bottom of all his troubles. When he finds this out he at once becomes a dangerous lunatic, liable at any time to acts of violence of a homicidal character. These patients belong to the most dangerous class with whom we have to deal, especially because of the retention of their intellectual faculties.[20]

Noyes believed that dangerousness was not so easily assessed. He suggested that in true paranoia the patients' behavior remained within the bounds that society would tolerate and that they did not require hospitalization. Noyes conceived of paranoia in terms of the continuum of paranoid states, from the "true paranoia" at the one pole and paranoid schizophrenia at the other extreme. Like Meyer, he suggested that interference and restraint was likely to complicate the condition by extending the delusional system and stimulating the hatred. He did not advise commitment unless the behavior was too disturbing socially or the patient became dangerous. He concluded:

If the paranoiac is considered dangerous, commitment, of course, becomes imperative. To determine when the paranoiac has actually become dangerous is not always easy. A careful evaluation of the patient's history will usually indicate the extent to which delusions may be expected to control behavior. If delusions have exerted an important influence on behavior and if they are directed toward particular individuals he should be considered dangerous. The character and intensity of his emotions will greatly aid in deciding the questions as to the hazard in the patient's liberty; the greater the hatred the more imperative his removal from society.[21]

Meyer, Peterson, White, and Noyes represent the essential beliefs of clinicians in predicting the dangerousness of the paranoiac. Some psychiatrists would have restrained the patient at any stage of the disease; other clinicians judged the ideational content, references to specific individuals, and the intensity of the emotions. These formulations did not change essentially over the next thirty years. The paranoiac remained the most uniformly and predictably dangerous lunatic in the psychiatric literature.[22]

### Emotional Insanity: Psychopathic Personality

The rise of medical criminology kept the idea of moral insanity alive. Although William Healy and Ben Karpman, for example, both explicitly rejected the existence of a specific criminal type who was only morally defective, they and others identified a class of "borderline types" whose psychiatric symptoms were of special interest to criminologists.[23]

Healy, Bernard Glueck, Sheldon Glueck, White, Strecker and Ebaugh, and Noyes in standard works of the first half of the twentieth century all identified this class of patients by the term "constitutional psychopathic inferiority" and later by the term "psychopathic personality." Like moral insanity, the idea remained inexact. Karpman organized a symposium at the Government Hospital for the Insane in 1923 to illuminate the concept. He summarized the predominant views: "In the psychopaths we have unstable individuals with marked volitional and temperamental [emotional], but not obviously intellectual defects."[24]

Psychopathic personalities were generally social nuisances rather than criminal lunatics. In 1934 the American Psychiatric Association specified that the term excluded intellectual and biological defects implied by the terms, "constitutional inferiority" and "constitutional defective." Attempts to classify various subtypes, such as Kraepelin's groups, were inadequate. Kraepelin, for example, had identified various types from 1896 on; in the next edition of his textbook, however, he modified the concept. In 1896 he had conceived of the psychopathic condition as "degeneracy insanity," namely, constitutional neurasthenia, compulsive insanity, impulsive insanity, psychic hermaphroditism, and homosexuality; in 1899 he included under this classification the born criminal, the unstable, the pathological liar and swindler, and pseudoligatory paranoiacs. Menninger noted that this classification introduced into psychiatry the concept of the born criminal, shaped by Lombroso. Other physicians' classifications of psychopathic personality included a wide variety of nonpsychotic conditions in which social maladjustment was the central diagnostic issue.[25]

By the turn of the century, the question of whether the intellect could remain intact in such a condition was largely put to rest. No longer was impaired reason an issue in psychiatric explanation. Noyes noted that, though more often psychopaths violated the conventions of society than they violated the law, the absence of any emotional restraint, or in dynamic terms, the failure of the superego, made these patients dangerous. Of the subtype "antisocial personality," Noyes contended in 1934:

These psychopaths show a moral and ethical blunting, a lack of sympathy for their fellow-men and a behavior destructive to the welfare of the social order. . . . Their emotional life is superficial and affectively cold. . . . Their offences may constitute the whole register of crime—theft, embezzlement, forgery, robbery, brutal sex attacks and other acts of violence. Many take pleasure in their struggle with the law and feel pride in their accomplishments. Punishments are considered as expressions of injustice and have no deterrent effect.[26]

Psychiatrists who were followers of Adolf Meyer tended to believe that such patients were constitutionally inferior. Rosanoff, for example, described the lack of remorse and the impulsiveness that characterized this class of psychopathic personalities. These characteristics led patients to acts of violence in order to satisfy their own desires without regard for the ethical consequences of such behavior.[27]

Psychiatrists recognized that, in the absence of moral restraint, the psychopathic personality could develop the symptoms of frank psychosis. These patients were dangerous and in need of restraint. Samuel Henry Kraines, of the University of Illinois College of Medicine, and a follower of Meyer as well, described a patient who was so unable or unwilling to control her behavior that Kraines recommended hospitalization and treated her with metrazol convulsive therapy. He stated in 1948: "If, for example, the patient is brutal, paranoid, with outbursts of dangerous rages, hospitalization is preferable to permitting such persons to be loose in society." The patient terrorized her family by "throwing dishes, coffee pots, and even knives at the family when in rage," which occurred at the least provocation when her demands were not met. Kraines stated, "In this patient none of the overt evidences of psychosis in the usual classification sense could be found, but her actions were obviously those which would not permit her to live in society."[28]

Psychiatrists associated the psychopathic personality with insane homicide. In 1934 N. S. Yawger, a neurologist at the Eastern (Pennsylvania) State Penitentiary, reported this case of a dangerous psychopath:

Jesse Pomeroy . . . perhaps spent more time—about 40 years—in solitary confinement than has any other prisoner in this country. His crimes began at 13 years and at 14 he was sentenced to life imprisonment and solitary confinement, only having escaped hanging by reason of his extreme youth. Within a few weeks he had stripped, trussed-up, beaten and otherwise tortured a number of little children. Because of these offenses he was detained in a reform school but good behavior procured his release after 17 months. Within the 2 months following, he tortured 2 more children, bruising, stabbing and mutilating them until they died. He made several unsuccessful attempts to escape from prison. While undergoing penal servitude tales were told of his continued cruelty and among other accusations was that of catching rats and skinning them alive.[29]

The predominant opinion in the psychiatric literature of the 'twenties and 'thirties was that the psychopathic personality was a menace to society and ought to be locked up. Dangerousness was positively associated with the excitable, unstable, and impulsive types, not only because of their tendencies toward uncontrollable and abusive behavior, but also because of their characteristic intelligent deviousness. These characteristics made these individuals unwelcome in the already troubled asylums. The consensus was that these types of patients were fit candidates for the penitentiary. They tended not to be identified in advance of their misdeeds, and so, though they were known to be dangerous, prevention was not a theme in the literature.[30]

## Homicidal Impulse (Obsessive-Compulsive Neurosis)

Throughout the nineteenth century, the existence of a "pure homicidal impulse" was a matter of controversy. By the end of the century, somatic alienists identified impulses, or imperative ideas, as a symptom of a variety of mental diseases, such as dementia praecox, constitutional psychopathic inferiority of hereditary or biological nature, and neurasthenia. Kraepelin identified "compulsive states" and "impulsive states" as symptoms of constitutional inferiority.[31] With the rise of dynamic psychiatry and the disengagement of the concept of psychopathic personality from hereditarian and biological deviation, impulses and imperative ideas became part of the broader category of psychoneuroses.

Sigmund Freud and Pierre Janet attenuated the impulse as a dangerous insanity. For Freud, the impulse was a symptom of obsessional neurosis. In 1917 Francis X. Dercum, of the Jefferson Medical College, cited Janet on the question of the dangerousness of the irresistible impulse: "Janet has strongly insisted on the absence of carrying out of the impulse. In over more than 200 cases, in which criminal impulses were present, he did not observe a single real occurrence, he did not observe a single crime committed nor a single suicide."[32] Like Janet, Dercum maintained that the impulse could be present and quite constant, but that it was not irresistible.

Psychoanalyst Ernest Jones, in his contribution to White and Jelliffe in 1913, maintained that the impulse, again not necessarily acted upon, was the principal diagnostic feature of the neurosis. He asserted, "The diagnostic feature of the neurosis, is the investment of various mental processes with a feeling of compulsions . . . as though the patient is being impelled against his will by an external force, and has lost normal control over his mental processes."[33] Jones reduced the symptoms to motor, sensory, ideational, and affective phenomena, but did not attribute any particular dangerousness to any of them.

Other dynamic psychiatrists, writing from the 'teens to the 'fifties, regarded imperative ideas as symptoms of neurosis. White in 1919 called impulsions and compulsions "disorders of volition," but he did not assign any predictive value to them.[34] Both White and Strecker and Ebaugh in 1935 posited dynamic explanations for these symptoms and recommended psychoanalytic treatment. Noyes's views on this issue was consistent with then current psychoanalytic theory: he did not assign any particular danger to "morbid impulses."[35]

Psychiatrists identified, however, a critical difference between the phenomenon of impulse proceeding from the imperative idea and the impulse arising out of psychotic thinking and in response to delusions and hallucinations. This latter phenomenon was also taken to be a symptom of incipient schizophrenia. Noyes noted that the neurotic patient suffered a strong conscious resistance to the obsessions and compulsions, but that schizophrenic patients could experience similar phenomena and not become particularly disturbed by them. Although the psychoneurotic was never considered dangerous, after 1950 psychiatrists wrote more frequently about the differential diagnosis of the pseudoneurotic schizophrenic whose homicidal impulses may not be benign.[36]

### Volitional Insanity: Epilepsy

It has already been shown that the dangerous epileptic was found more often in print than in clinical practice. Yet, warnings about these patients continued to occur in the psychiatric literature from 1910 to the 1980s. Healy, in his 1913 contribution to White and Jelliffe, maintained that, once the epileptic develops criminalistic tendencies, though Healy did not specify what these were, he "becomes at once from the standpoint of society a most dangerous fellow—his actions are so incalculable."[37]

The literature of epilepsy during the twenties and thirties presents a particularly confused understanding of a generally hopeless disease. Although some forms of it were distinctly associated with feeblemindedness and organic lesions, a wide range of other etiological explanations was made, including the conception of the disease as a "life-reaction disorder." Before the electroencephalogram demonstrated abnormal electric cerebral activity, in the absence of any demonstrable organic lesion, idiopathic epilepsy was particularly open to dynamic interpretation and psycho-therapeutic treatment.[38]

Psychiatrists continued to believe that epileptic patients acquired clinically identifiable personality traits that made them not only socially unwelcome, but also dangerous even in the absence of convulsions. Noyes, in 1934, described the epileptic personality in the pre-convulsive state: "As maturity is approached the earlier characteristics are accentuated and the patient is frequently an irritable, selfish, egotistic, impulsive, asocial, rigid personality with a considerable mixture of cruelty and sadism." Noyes conceded that not all epileptics were so unpleasant and suggested that the "so-called" epileptic makeup was a defensive reaction manifesting itself in the form of hypersensitivity, irritability, and egocentricity.[39]

One effect of the growth of dynamic psychiatry was a recognition of the relationship between the emotional stress of the environment and the epileptic personality and convulsions. One study in 1934 challenged "the popular conception of an inherited deteriorating personality as the underlying cause of epilepsy [which] has resulted in great misunderstanding and injustice to both the patient and his family." Edward M. Bridge, a neurologist, studied environmental influences upon the development of the peculiar traits of epileptic patients. He concluded that psychogenic factors contributed to epileptics' response to their convulsions and that these phenomena should be treated dynamically just as the physiological alteration that produced the cerebral dysfunctions were treated medically. Oskar Diethelm, of the New York Hospital, studied the relationship between emotional stress and convulsions and reported similar results. These and other dynamic psychiatrists suggested that the epileptic personality was a normal response to a degrading and hopeless illness.[40]

Ideas about the dangerousness of the epileptic did not go entirely unchallenged. In 1923 psychiatrist Harlan L. Paine reported a study of 200 epileptic patients who had been involuntarily committed to the Grafton (New Hamphire) State Hospital. Of these 200, only 53 were diagnosed, in the final analysis, as psychotic and they had been confined because they were dangerous. However, none of the 53 had committed homicide or any violence that had resulted in personal injury. Paine concluded that the epileptic personality and epileptic violence were exaggerated. In another study, the pathologist at the Binghamton (New York) State Hospital analyzed the clinical records of 200 cases of epileptic psychosis. Although ideas about the perceived dangerousness and lustful sexuality of these patients were expressed in the written records, none of them had been committed because of harming anyone.[41]

Two advances in the late 1930s changed psychiatrists' belief about epileptic dangerousness. The first advance was the use of clinical encephalography in diagnostic studies. The results of the first studies of 430 patients at the Emma Pendleton Bradley Home, in Providence, Rhode Island, in 1937 changed a number of concepts related to epilepsy. One immediate application of electroencephalography was to the study of delinquents. These findings reinforced beliefs about the biological basis for behavior.[42]

The second advance was the use of dilantin (phenitoin), an anticonvulsant drug that relieved or lessened seizures in countless patients. It was rapidly accepted in medical practice. Psychiatrists noted that, in addition to its anticonvulsant effects, the drug modified behavior in a significant number of patients.[43]

Histrionic references to the dangerousness of epileptics thereafter moderated gradually in the clinical literature. The belief that all of them were dangerous changed to the recognition that postictal homicide and dangerousness associated with the epileptic equivalents (psychomotor seizures, automatism, and *petit mal* status) were rare. Moreover, electroencephalographic studies of criminals has failed to demonstrate any statistical correlation between capital crimes and epilepsy.[44]

The idea of the constitutional epileptic personality as a source of dangerousness was finally put to rest as well. In 1941 a psychological study of epileptic patients undermined the concept. Psychologist M. F. Harrower-Erickson could find no evidence of intellectual deterioration or an epileptic personality. This study did, however, reaffirm the suggestions of the dynamic psychiatrists that the psychological impairments associated with epilepsy were the result of the lived-experience of the disease and not of any structural or somatic origin. Psychiatrists frequently cited this study in their writings thereafter.[45]

## New Theories and Old Predictors

The homicidal patients identified by psychiatrists and predictors of dangerousness discussed in the literature throughout this period, 1910–60, were the same as those that had prevailed throughout the nineteenth century. The theoretical explanations for dangerousness changed; dynamic psychiatrists posited new theories about the causes of insane homicide. But psychiatrists still identified potential dangerousness with the delusions of post-partum psychosis, paranoia, schizophrenia, imperative ideas, psychopathic personality, and temporal-lobe epilepsy. And psychiatrists continued to report cases of homicide connected with these specific psychiatric disorders.

The introduction of chlorpromazine and related drugs into the care of the psychotic patient between 1954 and 1960 brought about a radical change in the character of mental-health care. Psychotic episodes could be aborted and disorganized behavior brought under control. Two results were the reduction of the number of patients in mental hospitals and the shift from institutional to community psychiatry. More predictably dangerous patients were at large in the community and free to remain under medical supervision or to forgo treatment.

# 9

## Prediction, Confidentiality, and the Duty to Warn

After 1960 civil libertarians invaded the cloistered, stable world of ideas in American psychiatry. Physicians suddenly found that the concept of dangerousness in mental illness emerged as a prominent theoretical issue. When mental patients began to challenge the doctrine of *parens patriae*, the legal justification for involuntary commitment shifted from the need for treatment and the right of the state to impose it to the protection of society. The suddenly magnified standard of dangerousness as a test for commitability demonstrated the ambiguity of the concept. In the absence of explicit definition of the criterion of "dangerous to self or others," the difficulties of justly applying the diagnosis of dangerousness in practical situations became evident.

### Dangerousness and Involuntary Commitment

The American Bar Association undertook a study of state commitment statutes and published the findings in 1961. The study showed that, of thirty-seven jurisdictions, only five specified that the sole criterion for involuntary commitment was danger to self or others. Twelve other jurisdictions specified dangerousness as

120

one factor, but augmented their statutes with the doctrine of *parens patriae*.[1] None, however, defined dangerousness or how it was to be assessed.

A number of legal decisions throughout the 1960s called attention to the civil consequences of the diagnosis of dangerousness and the inadequacy of the diagnostic criteria. For example, Saleem A. Shah, chief of the Center for Studies of Crime and Delinquency, National Institute of Mental Health, identified fifteen decision points in the criminal-justice and mental-health systems where the criterion of dangerousness was applied in the absence of definition.[2] He and Alexander D. Brooks, professor of law at Rutgers University, specified the consequences of a diagnosis of dangerousness: (1) a lengthy, even indeterminate, involuntary confinement to a mental hospital; (2) in some states, transfer to a maximum-security hospital for the criminally insane, though the patient may not yet have committed any crime; (3) in some states, imprisonment rather than confinement in a hospital; (4) proof, usually by the patient, of nondangerousness as a condition of release.

Brooks's review of the legislative judicial, and medical attempts to define the concept showed that, as in the nineteenth and early twentieth century, dangerousness encompassed, in addition to physical injury to another person, minor violations of law, emotional injury, and injury to property. He concluded that psychiatric experts therefore supplied their own "idiosyncratic legal views, [their] personal set of values about the protection of persons and society, and [their] hidden agendas about appropriate dispositions of the mentally ill."[3]

Despite these theoretical defects, the trend toward using a standard of dangerousness continued; by 1974 twenty-nine states specified that the standard for involuntary commitment was "dangerous to self or others," but in none of these statutes was dangerousness defined.[4] Furthermore, the responsibility for making the diagnosis increasingly devolved upon the profession of psychiatry, which faced the problem of predicting dangerous behavior in unambiguous terms.

## The Search for Predictors

Because of this change in the laws, during the 1960s psychiatrists began to reconsider earlier studies on post-institutional dangerousness. These had done little to convince practitioners that mental patients were not dangerous and had little effect upon the problem of overcrowded mental hospitals. These traditional studies presented a number of methodological problems and left questions about the composition of research populations as well as the definition of dangerousness unanswered. Yet, it was noted in the 1970s, as before, that the results of such studies showed that released mental patients were no more dangerous to the community in terms of major crimes committed than was the general population.[5]

But other, and now new, studies of post-institutional dangerousness showed different results. In 1965 Jonas R. Rappeport and George Lassen, of the University of Maryland School of Medicine, studied populations of released mental patients by comparing arrest rates for serious crimes; their results showed that patients who had been diagnosed as schizophrenic and antisocial did in fact account for most cases of violent crime. Rappeport and Lassen believed, however, that no positive correlation existed between any diagnosed psychiatric disorder and dangerousness. They maintained that "arrests of ex-mental hospital patients were very largely concentrated in a relatively small, rather well-demarcated group of persons with previous criminal records, and their antisocial behavior was clearly correlated with well-known factors which operate in the general population and are not correlated with the factors of mental illness except in a negative way."[6]

Experts involved in the study of the problem of defining the concept of dangerousness posited alternate explanations for these positive findings.[7] Shah in 1978 suggested that the characteristics of persons being confined to mental hospitals had changed since 1960. In the studies conducted before that year, the populations under study had included patients who were never dangerous and some who, according to the investigators, were probably not even mentally ill. Shah suggested that current research demonstrated a positive correlation between previous and post-institutional dangerousness, not between psychiatric disorder and dangerousness.[8] Other authorities predicted an increase in the number of psychotic murders as a result of the release of unsupervised patients in the community; these previously dangerous patients might well be discharged and antipsychotic drugs prescribed for them, but it was not certain they would continue to take the medicine or avail themselves of the services of the community mental-health center. From these studies, however, psychiatrists reaffirmed the belief that the most reliable predictor of dangerousness was its previous existence.[9]

Research on such populations yielded little insight into the prediction of dangerousness in the absence of overt behaviors. In 1974 Henry J. Steadman, of the New York State Department of Mental Hygiene, a figure prominent in prediction research, established that no correlation was evident between assaultive behavior in a hospital and later in the community, an important consideration in discharge assessment. He suggested that patients in hospitals were removed from the situations that may precipitate dangerousness and might be receiving psychotropic drugs that modify the mental state. Moreover, he did not believe that any particular psychiatric disorder was a significant variable. Two major studies of large populations of patients transferred from maximum-security hospitals to civil hospitals confirmed his belief that neither clinical judgments nor statistical assessments of previous behaviors yielded any insight into the prediction of dangerousness; and the authors suggested that the scientific study of situational variables would be more fruitful.[10]

Studies of clinical predictions of dangerousness showed that they were usually based on clinical intuition rather than any specific methodology or psychiatric classification. One sociologist studied the social interaction among psychiatrist, psychologist, and psychiatric social worker teams appointed to reevaluate patients at the Lima (Ohio) State Hospital, a maximum security institution, in 1974. This study indicated that the diagnosis of

dangerousness or nondangerousness resulted from social interaction and the dominance of the psychiatrist in the group that appeared to be an apparently objective report.[11]

Another study demonstrated that psychiatrists did not use any
specific methodology in the prediction of dangerousness in sex
offenders. Under the 1963 California Mentally Disordered Sex
Offender Law, any offender believed to be mentally disordered,
convicted of a felony sex offense on a child under fourteen, and
having a prior similar conviction had to be assessed by psychiatrists in order to establish the diagnosis. Designation as a "mentally disordered sex offender" automatically carried with it the
diagosis of dangerousness. This study revealed that the psychiatrists relied upon the existence of previous criminal and social history rather than any clinical data or special methodology. The
psychological makeup of the subjects, all nonpsychotic sociopathic personalities, made the traditional mental-status examination useless. In the absence of overt psychiatric symptoms,
psychiatrists had only the statistical predictors to rely upon,
though an analysis of the narrative reports showed that the use of
the statistical predictor was unintentional.[12]

### Task Force 8: The Position of the Profession

By the end of the decade, the prediction of dangerousness had become central to the practice of psychiatry. The American Psychiatric Association appointed a task force to study the issue and
make recommendations. As a result of the comprehensive review
of all scientific data available, the task force concluded: "The
ability of psychiatrists or any other professionals to reliably predict future violence is unproved."[13] Yet, within the context of
the report and the medical literature of the 1970s, the profession
continued to associate predictable dangerousness with particular
psychiatric disorders and mental phenomena. In the absence of a
reliable methodology that would permit practitioners to predict
on the basis of situational variables, they used the only one available to them.

### Psychiatric Disorder and Clinical Dangerousness

Despite the task force's conclusion that psychiatrists overpredicted dangerousness, not all practitioners agreed with the task force that dangerousness could not in any circumstance be predicted.[14] The task force had, in fact, identified the characteristics of insane homicide and of the violent patient, the same ones Ray had specified in 1838.[15]

One critical feature of the report was the application of the situation-based model. The task-force psychiatrists posited that violence was the function of the psychiatric disorder and the patient's lived-experience. According to the task force: "Violent patients are seldom randomly or irrationally violent but respond with violence . . . to dynamically significant stresses and situations."[16] The position of the task-force was therefore that dangerousness could not be predicted because the future social situation of the patient could not be assessed.

Although the task-force members maintained that no positive association existed between clinical diagnosis and crimes of violence, they identified three classes of patients who were theoretically capable of violence: (1) overtly psychotic patients who had delusions and hallucinations; (2) the antisocial explosive or passive-aggressive personality types; and (3) victims of brain dysfunction, such as epilepsy.[17]

The task force also identified predictors of dangerousness that could be elicited in the course of the mental-status examination: "Delusional patients with violent fantasies should be taken seriously." It was also recognized that individuals reporting homicidal impulses might be in a state of incipient psychosis. Although patients may be anxious about losing control, a characteristic of obsessive-compulsive neurosis, the task force stated: "Certain more schizoid or obsessive patients may report violent urges in a clinically detached way. . . . The calmness of these patients is defensive. . . . Patients with personality disorders such as those of the Explosive, Antisocial, or Passive-aggressive types must be asked questions about past acts of violence as they are apt to reveal little overt psychopathology."[18] These assertions about the dangerousness of certain mental disorders are consistent with the findings of nineteenth- and twentieth-century authorities.

The belief that certain psychiatric disorders were positively associated with insane homicide was evident in the textbooks published throughout the 1970s. Although the rhetoric was subtle compared to that in earlier generations, the connection was still clear. For example, in reference to paranoia in 1940 Strecker asserted, "All cases of paranoia should be committed since they are always potentially dangerous." Kolb stated in the eighth edition of *Modern Clinical Psychiatry* (1973): "Among common causes for the commitment of paranoid patients are homicidal and suicidal attempts, the writing of anonymous letters to persons in authority, litigation, or persistent statements that they are victims of conspiracy."[19] In the second edition of the *American Handbook of Psychiatry* (1974), Sandor Rado wrote: "But if a paranoid acts out publicly his aggression, which to him seems justified and completely reasonable, he is usually met by some social sanction."[20] Freedman, Kaplan, and Sadock, in the second edition of *Modern Synopsis of Comprehensive Textbook of Psychiatry/II* (1976), suggested that "occasionally, the paranoid person turns his hostility against his persecutor and makes either verbal or physical attacks on others."[21] Other major textbooks of the decade did not specify any predictable dangerousness associated with paranoia.[22]

These medical writers generally recognized the relationship between morbid impulses and incipient schizophrenia that was identified in the task-force report. Although psychiatric textbooks specified that the impulses of obsessive-compulsive neurosis were not dangerous, the further idea that they could be dangerous when unaccompanied by anxiety was usually excluded. Writers did, however, describe the process of differential diagnosis in morbid impulse. They specified that this impulse could be diagnostic of incipient schizophrenia, but they did not state plainly that it could make the patient dangerous.[23]

Psychiatrists still confronted the issue of insane homicide in schizophrenia. Freedman, Kaplan, and Sadock state: "It is exceedingly difficult to prevent most schizophrenic homicides, since usually there is no clear warning. The homicidal schizophrenic patient may appear to be relaxed, even apathetic—then, within a day or two, he kills somebody. . . . The most significant single factor in many suicides and homicides is a traumatic experience of rejection."[24]

Most psychiatrists referred to both the unpredictability and the rarity of homicide in schizophrenia. Day and Semrad, in the *Harvard Guide to Modern Psychiatry* (1978), wrote: "Although catatonics and enraged paranoids may be violent, homicide is rare. Lehmann . . . attributed both suicide and homicide to the schizophrenic's profound sensitivity to rejection by a figure on whom he relies." Lehmann said further: "The number of homicides committed by schizophrenics may increase during the next few years. As a result of the gradual reduction in hospital confinement of schizophrenics, many of them are treated with modern methods of therapy in the community, where it is often impossible to control and supervise their pharmacotherapy and to prevent recurrence of paranoid homicidal behavior."[25]

The potential dangerousness of patients continued to be identifed with personality disorders. Of persons with sociopathic personality, Kolb in 1973 asserted, "When frustrated, they may be dangerous to others. Their offenses may constitute the whole register of crime—theft, embezzlement, forgery, robbery, brutal sex attacks, and other acts of violence."[26]

Psychiatrists believed that the sociopathic patient was capable of the most bizarre acts of insane homicide. MacDonald reported the following case: "One psychopathic murderer drove around for several days with the dead body of his victim in the trunk of his car. A girl friend inquired about the smell coming from the back of his car, and he replied with considerable aplomb that it was a crate of limburger cheese. Eventually the smell became sufficient to arouse the curiosity of the police, thus leading to the suspect's arrest."[27] MacDonald believed that the source of dangerousness in this psychiatric disorder was the absence of moral restraint and the inability to experience remorse.

Finally, the connection between epilepsy and dangerousness was still acknowledged. With the development of computerized axial tomography and stereotactic surgical techniques, not only had cortical function become better understood, but also the function of the inaccessible neural structures. Many clinicians believed that stereotaxic electroencephalograms of the amygdala and depth electrode stimulation supported the validity of the observations of ninteenth-century alienists concerning *mania transitoria* and the occurrence of homicide in epilepsy. Although the existence of the epileptic personality had been challenged, neurological and psychological studies of epileptics with personality disorders demonstrated to the investigators' satisfaction that the personality constellation described by these earlier observers is positively associated with temporal-lobe epilepsy.[28]

Physicians of the 1970s and 1980s commonly associate pathology of the amygdala with violent behavior. In a widely cited work, Mark, Sweet, and Ervin, of the Harvard Medical School, using stereotaxic electrode technology, recorded the electrical activity of the brain during violent episodes in temporal-lobe epilepsy and, through electrical stimulation of the amygdala, produced violent behavior in patients with temporal-lobe epilepsy.[29]

### Psychiatric Emergencies

Practitioners' beliefs about the prediction of dangerousness were most clearly articulated in the literature of psychiatric emergencies. Despite the acknowledgment that the situational variables in any case make future dangerousness unpredictable, the psychiatrist or other physician must make such clinical judgments in emergencies on the basis of inadequate data.[30] And, though the task force report had warned that "psychiatric expertise in the prediction of 'dangerousness' is not established and clinicians should avoid 'conclusory' judgments in this regard," it also recognized that in emergencies the clinician had to make a judgment:[31] "Decision-making in this difficult area requires specifying the degree of immediate risk and the type of risk which the patient presents to others."[32]

A survey of the literature on psychiatric emergencies from 1972 to the early 1980s shows that the predictors of dangerousness most commonly identified were: (1) command hallucinations directed toward killing another person (catatonic schizophrenia, schizo-phrenic reactions); (2) delusions whose content was related to kill-ing another person (paranoia, paranoid schizophrenia); (3) morbid impulses without anxiety (incipient schizophrenia, decompen-sating obsessive-compulsive neurosis); (4) episodic behavior dys-control (temporal-lobe epilepsy, explosive personality); and finally, though usually not seen in an emergency room but in con-nection with criminal behavior, (5) personality disorder (socio-pathic personality). These writers acknowledged the role of drugs, alcohol, organic states, interpersonal stress, and social malad-justment in producing these phenomena. When the behavior was attributed to nonpsychiatric conditions, physicians advised that the patient should be discharged to the care of family and friends. When the behavior could be traced to psychiatric disorder, in-voluntary commitment was recommended if the patient was un-able to agree willingly to hospitalization.[33]

In 1976 the problem of dangerous insanity and its prediction assumed a new dimension and redefined the therapeutic relation-ship between the homicidal insane and all primary mental-health professionals. Prosenjit Poddar was a patient of a clinical psy-chologist at Cowell Hospital, in Berkeley, a University of Cali-fornia institution. In August 1969 Poddar told the therapist that he intended to kill Tatiana Tarasoff, his former girl friend. The therapist requested that the campus police detain his patient, but he appeared rational so he was soon released. The therapist then wrote to the civil police requesting the man's confinement, but the chief psychiatrist countermanded this decision. On October 27, 1969, when Miss Tarasoff returned to the United States, Poddar murdered her.[34]

The parents sued the therapists, the police, and the regents of the University of California for failing to confine the man under the state's commitment law and to warn their daughter of the dan-ger. The defendants claimed that they had no duty to warn. The court found for them, and the plaintiffs appealed. The California Supreme Court held for the plaintiffs on the basis of foreseeability and contended that a special relationship existed between the par-ties. Furthermore, the court found that the need for public safety prevailed over the confidential therapeutic relationship. Both courts acknowledged the theoretical difficulties of predicting dangerousness, but Poddar's therapist had already done so.

The precedent set by the *Tarasoff* decision was absolute only in California. But, within the last decade, several additional courts have embraced the rationale. Mental-health professionals objected that the ruling required a breach of confidentiality, and in view of the difficulties in predicting dangerousness, combined now with the legal sanctions for failure to predict, would lead to disruption of the therapeutic process. Nevertheless, mental-health professionals recognize the duty to protect the victim of the homicidal insane.[35]

After 1960 the care of the psychiatric patient was no longer the exclusive province of the medical profession. Advances in treatment and changes in the social context shifted care from the hospital to the community. Patients challenged the doctrine of *parens patriae*, and the prediction of dangerousness emerged as the primary, and in some states the only, criterion for involuntary commitment. Ironically, the sanctions against such commitment impeded action in the case of Prosenjit Poddar, which led to a landmark court decision that further complicated the care of the homicidal insane. Still, the concept of dangerousness and its prediction became a prominent theoretical, legal, and social issue.

# The Phenomenology of  10
# Homicidal Insanity

From the beginning of the nineteenth century to the 1980s, physicians believed that mental disorder could make people dangerous. At first, insane homicide was associated with insanity as a unitary disease; then, as a more critical clinical empiricism evolved, the profession associated homicide with only certain types of disorders. Although notions about the essential nature of mental illness changed amid the scientific and cultural changes over the past two centuries, doctors have maintained a remarkable intersubjective agreement about homicidal insanity.

Throughout almost two hundred years, psychiatrists conceived of mental disorder as having predominantly intellectual, emotional, or volitional features. The early classifications of the French and British clinicians were squarely founded upon a faculty psychology. After this idea waned, psychiatric thinkers continued to organize the critical features of disorders in this way. Therefore, it is possible to trace certain concepts from 1800 to the present using this framework.

## Intellectual Insanity

By 1800 physicians had noted that people who committed insane homicide sometimes did so under the influence of delusions and command hallucinations. They referred to this phenomenon as delusional insanity, but tended to identify puerperal mania as a separate entity, though in many instances the disorder was characterized by delusions and hallucinations. Esquirol, in 1828, called delusional insanity "intellectual monomania"; and, though this remained the most commonly used term over the next sixty years, others employed "homicidal mania" and "delusional insanity." By 1860 physicians had identified the "homicidal crank" as predictably dangerous. These patients were usually troublesome individuals whose delusions were reinforced by the cirsumstances they created in their daily lives.

During the 1880s the concept of monomania as homicidal insanity underwent theoretical change, but the belief that delusions and command hallucinations were predictors of dangerousness did not. The German neurophysiologists introduced the term *Primäre Veruchtheit* to designate a condition in which the sole mental symptom was delusions of persecution; Richard von Krafft-Ebing used the term "paranoia" to designate the phenomenon. English-speaking physicians rapidly adopted the latter.

Many psychiatrists continued to believe that delusions were the principal, if not the sole, cause of insane homicide. Most patients who committed homicide under the influence of delusions and command hallucinations were not brought to trial. However, throughout the nineteenth century, cases were reported in the literature of insane patients who were executed for homicide despite the predominance of delusions and hallucinations and despite the influence of expert medical testimony.

By the end of the nineteenth century, Kraepelin's clinical description and classification of mental disorders began to be used in the United States. Alienists considered delusions and hallucinations to be part of the complicated symptomatology of dementia praecox. Although Adolf Meyer had suggested a dynamic interpretation of this disease in 1909, Eugen Bleuler's similarly dynamic interpretation modified the concept into schizophrenia. By 1930 psychiatrists wrote more about the dynamics of schizophrenia in their textbooks and papers than the prediction of dangerousness. Nevertheless, it was believed that the delusions, hallucinations, and senseless impulsivity of schizophrenia made these patients dangerous. After the 1950s less was written about their dangerousness, but the predictors have remained the same to the present time.

Psychiatrists came to recognize that paranoia as a pure disorder of the intellect was rare. After 1910 they tended to think in terms of a continuum of paranoid "states," in which a subclinical form was at one extreme and the frank psychosis of paranoid schizophrenia at the other. Still, belief in the potential dangerousness of the paranoid patient did not change.

### Emotional Insanity

Pinel, in 1801, and Rush, in 1812, both described insane behavior they believed was caused by derangement of the emotional faculty. They contended that the intellect could remain unaffected in certain forms of insanity, an idea debated throughout the nineteenth century. Esquirol differentiated between emotional insanity (*manie sans délire*) and volitional insanity (variously called irresistible impulse, homicidal impulse, and homicidal monomania throughout the nineteenth century). By 1835 Prichard had described moral insanity, which at first included both the emotional and volitional insanities. In 1842 he modified the concept and defined moral insanity as a disorder of the emotions. Like Esquirol, he conceived of the insane impulse as a disorder of volition.

From 1840 until the start of the twentieth century, some physicians rejected the existence of moral insanity as a psychiatric disorder because they believed that the intellect could not remain unaffected in any insanity. Yet, reported cases characterized morally insane persons as possessing devious intelligence in the absolute absence of moral restraint. The clinical literature described morally insane, yet intellectually intact, patients who committed gruesome homicides, often preceded by rape and torture of the victims. By the turn of the twentieth century, however, the controversy over whether or not the intellect could remain intact in insanity had been put to rest.

The term "moral insanity" predominated in the literature until the 1880s, when the idea that the lack of moral feelings or restraint was a stigmatum of atavistic degeneration changed the concept. Such terms as "degenerative moral imbecility" and, a few years later, "constitutional psychopathic inferiority" were most commonly used to designate the psychopathy phenomenon. Kraepelin was the first to use the term "psychopathic personality," which continued in common use until the 1950s. By then, the idea that the causes originated in the environment and not in the biology of the patient, a position maintained by dynamic psychiatrists and criminologists, had gained status; and the term was changed to "sociopathic personality." Kraepelin also initiated the positive association of criminality with the sociopathic personality that has prevailed throughout the twentieth century. Physicians have believed from 1800 to the present that the absence of moral feelings, "conscience," or the emotion of remorse is a predictor of insane homicide.

### Impulsive Insanity

Both Pinel and Rush described morbid impulses, and Esquirol named the the one to kill as "homicidal monomania." Not all physicians believed that morbid impulses were insanity. As in the debate over the issue of moral insanity, some pointed to the primacy of intellectual functioning. But, throughout the 19th century, cases of homicidal impulse were reported in the medical literature.

By the end of that century, the homicidal impulse, and impulses in general, came to be regarded as a symptom of psychiatric illness rather than as a primary disorder. Kraepelin suggested that the morbid impulse was a symptom of incipient dementia praecox; he described the impulse to kill in the absence of apparent involvement of the intellect, which was characterized by an emotional detachment from the gravity of the crime. These observations explained the enigma of the Cornier case, for example, and the case reported by Wigglesworth in 1901, in which both patients decapitated their victims under the influence of a morbid impulse, emotional indifference, and clear intellect.

Neuropsychiatrists after 1880 believed that the morbid impulse was a sign of a weakened and/or degenerate nervous system, an idea supported by the hereditarian and environmental theories prevalent before 1900. Kraepelin believed that the morbid impulse, in addition to incipient dementia praecox, reflected constitutional inferiority. In 1917 Freud described the obsessional neurosis as a benign condition in which the patient suffered from imperative ideas but did not act upon them. Dynamic psychiatrists followed Freud in their contention that the obsessive-compulsive neurosis, as it came to be called in twentieth-century classifications, though making patients suffer greatly, did not make them dangerous.

Psychiatrists recognized, however, that the morbid impulses of incipient schizophrenia were predictors of dangerousness. After 1940 the literature emphasized the differential diagnosis of the suffering psychoneurotic and the emotionally indifferent pseudoneurotic schizophrenic whose morbid impulses may not be benign.

## Volitional Insanity

By 1800 physicians had observed cases of insanity that they believed were a primary disorder of volition, usually designated by the term "mania." Undoubtedly, this designation included cases of what Kraepelin later described as the manic phase of manic-depressive psychosis, but by the 1830s these patients were considered to be dangerous because of the frank delusions and hallucinations with mania. Physicians suggested that epileptics were subject to attack of a similar type, epileptic mania or "furor," which occurred before, after, or in place of the *grand mal* seizure. Accordingly, epileptics were greatly feared by physicians and the general public as the most uniformly and predictably dangerous patient known to medicine. By the 1870s physicians began to describe the "interparoxysmal mental state," or the so-called epileptic personality, that made the patient dangerous in the absence of seizures. These ideas persisted up until the late 1930s despite extensive clinical evidence that few of these patients were dangerous.

In the 1850s some physicians accepted a new idea that a person could experience a state of transitory frenzy (despite the absence of any neuropathology and that the state could abate completely within a few hours or days. Although the idea of *mania transitoria* was lent credence by the rise of dynamic neurophysiology after 1860, the clinical evidence to support the existence of the disorder was scarce, and so, by the end of the nineteenth century, physicians believed that the phenomenon was associated with epilepsy.

As the electroencephalogram and refined stereotaxic techniques for studying the electrophysiology of the cortical and subcortical structures became available, researchers conducted experiments on human subjects that led to conclusions paralleling the observations of the early nineteenth-century physicians. Electrical derangement of the amygdala produced a transitory state that was akin to the descriptions of *mania transitoria* and epileptic furor. Twentieth-century neurophysiologists thus confirmed that patients with temporal-lobe epilepsy can be dangerous.

Throughout almost two centuries, the prediction of dangerousness and the prevention of insane homicide have been predominant themes in the practice of psychiatry. But, before 1960, practitioners, protected by the doctrine of *parens patriae*, were only rarely required to predict dangerousness as a criterion for involuntary commitment. The principal application of any prediction technique was in the matter of management of patients in the asylum and their release. Then, in the 1960s, involuntary commitment became a civil-rights issue. In many states, the sole criterion became "danger to self or others." Since the 1976 landmark Tarasoff ruling, psychiatrists are being held responsible for predicting dangerousness and, furthermore, for taking steps to protect potential victims of the homicidal insane. In response, the American Psychiatric Association has taken the position that dangerousness cannot be predicted and maintained that this concept in insanity has never been adequately defined.

Nevertheless, proof of dangerousness to self or others is increasingly being made the standard for involuntary hospitalization. Statutory definitions of mental illness are becoming more precise in language, and commitment based upon dangerousness requires, more and more, specific proof of overt threats or acts. Several courts have ruled that evidence indicating a patient suffers from a mental disorder in which insane homicide is known to occur is insufficient. Generally, in the absence of overt threats or acts, the prediction of dangerousness based upon clinical facts must be clear and persuasive. The prediction and prevention of insane homicide continues to this day to be a complex human scientific problem—and perhaps an unresolvable dilemma.

# Notes

## Chapter 1: The Issue of Insane Homicide

1. Alvin M. Mesnikoff and Carl G. Lauterbach, "The Association of Violent Dangerous Behavior with Psychiatric Disorders: A Review of the Research Literature," *Journal of Psychiatry and Law*, 3 (1975), 415–46. See also Alan A. Stone, *Mental Health and Law: A System in Transition* (Rockville, Maryland, 1975), 27–28; American Psychiatric Association, *Task Force Report* 8: Clinical Aspects of the Violent Individual (Washington, D.C., 1974); and American Psychiatric Association, *Diagnostic and Statistical Manual of Mental Disorders*, 3rd ed. (Washington, D.C., 1980).
2. Karl Menninger, *The Vital Balance: The Life Process in Mental Health and Illness* (New York, 1963). In the early literature, for example, physicians used the words mania, melancholia, and delirium to describe a number of different disorders and mental phenomena. Early psychiatrists attempted to devise classifications based upon faculty psychology or upon the natural course of the disease.
3. Gerald N. Grob, *Mental Illness and American Society, 1875–1940* (Princeton, New Jersey, 1873), 7–29.
4. Thomas S. Szasz, *Law, Liberty, and Psychiatry: An Inquiry into the Social Uses of Mental Health Practices* (New York, 1963), 229. See also Szasz, *Psychiatric Slavery* (New York, 1977); and David Ingleby, ed., *Critical Psychiatry: The Politics of Mental Health* (New York, 1980).

## Chapter 2: The Theoretical Boundaries of Dangerousness, 1800—1840

1. For an analysis of the social changes during the Colonial and early National periods that affected the status of the mentally ill, see Albert Deutsch, *The*

*Mentally Ill in America: A History of Their Care and Treatment from Colonial Times,* 2nd ed. (New York, 1949), 39–71; Gerald N. Grob, *Mental Institutions in America: Social Policy to 1875* (New York, 1973), 1–34; Norman Dain, *Concepts of Insanity in the United States, 1789–1865* (New Brunswick, New Jersey, 1964), 1–52; Leland V. Bell, *Treating the Mentally Ill from Colonial Times to the Present* (New York, 1980), 1–14; and Andrew T. Scull, "The Discovery of the Asylum Revisited: Lunacy Reform in the New American Republic," in Scull, ed., *Madhouses, Mad-Doctors, and Madmen: The Social History of Psychiatry in the Victorian Era* (Philadelphia, 1981), 144–65.

2. Dain, *Disordered Minds: The First Century of Eastern State Hospital in Williamsburg, Virginia, 1766–1866,* (Charlottesville, Virginia, 1971), 7–8; Virginia *Gazette* (Purdie and Dixon), July 6, 1769; Virginia *Gazette* (Purdie and Dixon), November 5, 1772.

3. Deutsch, *The Mentally Ill in America,* 1949 ed., 158–212. See also Merle Curti, *The Growth of American Thought* (New York, 1943), 169–72.

4. Bayle, *Recherches sur les malades mentales* (Paris, 1822). For a summary of the influence of French clinical medicine upon medical education and practice in the United States, see John Duffy, *The Healers: A History of American Medicine* (Chicago, 1979), 98–108. See also Francis R. Packard, *History of Medicine in the United States* (New York, 1963), 2, 951–1051; Fielding H. Garrison, *An Introduction to the History of Medicine,* 4th ed. (Philadelphia, 1929), 407–20; and Richard H. Schryock, *Medicine and Society in America, 1660–1860* (New York, 1960), 12–32.

5. Parkman, *Proposals for Establishing a Retreat for the Insane* (Boston, 1814), 4.

6. Russel Blaine Nye, *Society and Culture in America, 1830–1860* (New York, 1974), 331–33. See also Thomas C. Upham, *Elements of Intellectual Philosophy* (Boston, 1827). Upham's text was revised numerous times and was still in print in 1886.

7. Pinel, *A Treatise on Insanity,* trans. D. D. Davis (London 1806), 92–93.

8. *Ibid.,* 142, 172, 204.

9. *Ibid.,* 142, 152.

10. *Ibid.,* 155.

11. Beck, *Inaugural Dissertation on Insanity,* (New York, 1811), 28.

12. *Ibid.,* 32.

13. Rush, *Medical Inquiries and Observations upon the Diseases of the Mind,* 2nd ed. (Philadelphia, 1818), 181–83. See also Dain, *Concepts of Insanity,* 183. For a summary of Rush's beliefs about the moral faculty, see Eric T. Carlson and Meribeth M. Simpson, "Benjamin Rush's Medical Use of the Moral Faculty," *Bulletin of the History of Medicine,* 39 (1965), 22–23.

14. Carlson and Simpson, "Benjamin Rush's Medical Use of the Moral Faculty," 264. See also Rush, *Medical Jurisprudence* (Philadelphia, 1810).

15. Parkman, *Proposals,* 8–12.

16. Beck, *Elements of Medical Jurisprudence,* 3rd ed. (London, 1829), 230.

17. *Ibid.,* 248.

18. *Dictionary of American Biography* (New York, 1929), 2, 116–17. See also Samuel D. Gross, ed., *Lives of Eminent American Physicians and Surgeons of the Nineteenth Century* (Philadelphia, 1861), 776–79.

19. Georget, *Discussion médico-légale sur la folie* (Paris, 1826); Esquirol *Des maladies*

*mentales* (Paris, 1828); Esquirol, *Observations on the Illusions of the Insane and upon the Medico-Legal Question of Their Confinement*, trans. William Liddell (London, 1833); Prichard, *A Treatise on Insanity and Other Disorders Affecting the Mind* (London, 1835).

20. Conolly, *An Inquiry Concerning the Indications of Insanity with Suggestions for the Better Protection and Care of the Insane* (1830), facsimile reprint (London, 1964), 341.
21. *Ibid.*, 340.
22. *Ibid.*, 339.
23. *Ibid.*, 455–69.
24. *Ibid.*, 444–49.
25. *Ibid.*, 454.
26. Conolly, *The Treatment of the Insane without Mechanical Restraints* (London, 1856), 44.
27. Prichard, *A Treatise on Insanity and Other Disorders Affecting the Mind* (London, 1835:) Prichard, *A Treatise on Diseases of the Nervous System. Part the First. Comprising Convulsive and Maniacal Affections* (London, 1822). See also *The Dictionary of National Biography* (London, 1921–22), 16, 345.
28. Prichard, *Treatise on Insanity.* See also Esquirol, *Des maladies mentales*, 346; Eric T. Carlson and Norman Dain, "The Meaning of Moral Insanity," *Bulletin of the History of Medicine*, 36 (1962), 130–40; and M. K. Amdur, "Jean-Étienne Dominique Esquirol: His work and Importance for Modern Psychiatry," *American Journal of Psychiatry*, 18 (1939), 129–35.
29. Prichard, *Treatise on Insanity*, 386.
30. *Ibid.*, 380. See also Roger Smith, *Trial by Medicine: Insanity and Responsibility in Victorian Trials* (Edinburgh, 1981), 37. Up until this point, the sole judicial criterion in English and Continental courts for exculpable insanity was the existence of delusion.
31. Prichard, *Treatise on Insanity*, 112. See also Carlson and Dain, "The Meaning of Moral Insanity," 130–40.
32. Esquirol, *Des maladies mentales*, 320, 362.
33. Prichard, *On the Different Forms of Insanity in Relation to Jurisprudence* (London, 1842), 19.
34. Georget, *Discussion médico-légale*, 16. See also J. L. Michu, *Discussion médico-légale, la monomanie homicide, a propos du muertre commis par Henriette Cornier* (Paris, 1826), 33–39; and C. C. H. Marc, *De la folie, considérée dans ses rapports avec les questions médico-judiciares. Tome Deuxième* (Paris, 1840), 86.

"Henriette Cornier, femme Bretonne, aged 27 years, domestic servant, was of mild and lively disposition, always full of gaiety and vivacity, and remarkably fond of children. In the month of June, 1825, a singular change was observed in her character: she became silent, melancholy, absorbed on reverie, and was soon dismissed from her service. She fell gradually into a permanent stupor. Her friends were alarmed, suspected that she was pregnant, but were mistaken: they could never obtain from her any account of the cause of her dejection, though she was frequently interrogated. In the month of September she made an attempt to drown herself in the Seine, but was prevented.

In the following October the relatives of H. Cornier procured her another employment at the house of Dame Fournier. The change of condition made no abatement in her dejection and profound melancholy.

On the 4th of November, the conduct of Henriette Cornier not having been previously in any way different from her usual behavior, she suddenly conceived and immediately executed the act for which she was committed.

About noon, Dame Fournier went from home and told H. Cornier to prepare dinner, and to go to a neighboring shop, kept by Dame Belon, to buy some cheese. Henriette had always caressed a beautiful little girl, nineteen months old, the child of Belon. On this day she went to the shop and displayed the greatest fondness for the little girl, and persuaded Dame Belon, who was at first rather unwilling, to let her take it out for a walk. H. Cornier immediately took the child with her to the house of Dame Fournier, then empty, mounted to the common staircase with a large knife which she took from the kitchen, and stretching the child across the bed, with one stroke cut off its head. The head, which she held in her hand, she placed by the casement, and then put the body on the floor near to it. All these proceedings occupied about a quarter of an hour; during this time Henriette Cornier remained perfectly calm: she experienced no emotion of any kind. Dame Belon presently came to seek her child, and called Henriette, from the bottom of the stairs. 'What do you want?' said the latter, advancing on the ascending stairs. 'Your child is dead!' replied Henriette, with perfect coolness. Belon, alarmed, became more earnest; and Henriette again pronounced the words, 'Il est mort votre enfant!' As Belon forced her way into the room, Henriette took the child's head from the casement, and threw it by the open window into the street. The mother rushed out of the house, struck with horror. An alarm was raised; the father of the child and officers of justice with a crowd of persons entered. Henriette was found sitting on a chair near the body of the child, gazing at it, with the bloody knife by her, her hands and clothes covered with blood. She made no attempt for a moment to deny the crime; confessed all the circumstances, even her premeditated design and the perfidy of her caresses, which had persuaded the unhappy mother to entrust to her the child. It was found impossible to excite in her the slightest emotion of remorse or grief; to all that was said she replied, with indifference, "J'ai voulu le tuer! [I chose to kill it!]' " Marc, *De la folie*, 86.

35. Ray, *A Treatise on the Medical Jurisprudence of Insanity* (Boston, 1838), 50.
36. *Ibid.*, 96, 122, 137, 168.
37. *Ibid.*, 122.
38. *Ibid.*, 102, 104.
39. *Ibid.*, 126.
40. *Ibid.*, 139.
41. Smith, *Trial by Medicine*, 40–56. Smith suggests that this montage of physicalist theories was an expression of the ideal of *Naturwissenschaft*, and, for medical men, "physicalism was the intellectual means for coupling their necessarily mundane practice with the ideals of a new age." (p.41)
42. Ray, *Medical Jurisprudence*, 185–95.
43. For a concise biographical sketch and analysis of Ray's development as an alienist, see Jacques M. Quen's Introduction to Ray, *Contributions to Mental Pathology* (1873), facsimile reprint (Delmar, New York, 1973), v–x.

44. Dain, *Concepts of Insanity*, 62–66. See also John D. Davis, *Phrenology, Fad and Science: A* 19th Century American Crusade (New Haven, Connecticut, 1955); and Eric T. Carlson, "The Influence of Phrenology on Early American Psychiatric Thought," *American Journal of Psychiatry*, 115 (1958), 535–38. For an essay on the various editions of Spurzheim's published writings, see Anthony Walsh's Introduction to Spurzheim's *Observations on the Deranged Manifestations of the Mind, or Insanity* (London, 1817). Charles H. Steadman edited the second American edition of Spurzheim, *The Anatomy of the Brain with a General View of the Nervous System*, trans. R. Willis (Boston, 1836). This work is a descriptive neuroanatomy. Steadman was then surgeon at the United States Marine Hospital.

45. Carlson, "The Influence of Phrenology on Early American Psychiatric Thought," 535. See also Gerald N. Grob, "Samuel Woodward and the Practice of Psychiatry in Early Nineteenth-Century America," *Bulletin of the History of Medicine*, 36 (1962), 423–24.

46. Dain, *Concepts of Insanity*, 61–62, 80–81. See also Curti, *The Growth of American Thought*, 236; and Curti, *Human Nature in American Thought* (Madison, Wisconsin, 1980), 164–65. Despite an apparent internal contradiction between the metaphysical idea of unity of soul and the materialistic source of knowledge or moral behavior, Brigham, Ray and John Gray, for example, were able to reconcile the correspondence of spirit and matter in the Cartesian manner. See Dain's discussion of this contradiction, 61–63.

47. Esquirol, *Des maladies mentales*, 471–74. Esquirol reviewed the clinical investigations on craniometry and drew conclusions about the coincidence of the volume and form of the brain with intellectual capacity. "For those who are fond of this kind of investigations [*sic*], I subjoin a table of the mean results of admeasurements of the head, taken from women in the enjoyment of good health, and from plaster casts, taken after death, in the case of 36 insane women, 17 imbeciles, and 17 idiots." The figures showed some variations among the measurements of three classes of subjects. Esquirol concluded: "That if we suppose, that the sum of these four admeasurements, express the volume of the brain; it follows that the volume of this organ, diminishing in the same proportion with the intellectual capacity; that the cranium, would be the expression of this capacity." 474.

48. Spurzheim, *Phrenology, or the Doctrine of Mental Phenomena* (Boston, 1832), 143. See especially Ray's discussion of neuropathology in *Medical Jurisprudence*, 134–39. See also Dain, *Concepts of Insanity*, 60.

49. Spurzheim, *Phrenology*, 147.

50. Ibid., 60, 61. Spurzheim's argument was that the propensity to kill was innate and served a useful purpose for human existence; he said, "The God of Israel was fond of blood-shedding, and without it there was no remission of sin." 146. See also Dain, *Concepts of Insanity*, 82–83.

51. Spurzheim, *Phrenology*, 63.

52. Ibid., 245–46.

53. Combe, *Observations on Mental Derangement: Being an Application of the Principles of Phrenology to the Elucidation of the Causes, Symptoms, Nature, and Treatment of Insanity* (Boston, 1834), 229.

54. Ibid.. Combe returned to an earlier idea of congestion of blood in the brain

as the basic neuropathological mechanism. The cause of the irresistible impulse was to be "sought in congestion of blood to the brain." By this time, the discovery of the neurovascular bundle supported the theory that an intimate balance existed between the blood supply and the function of nervous tissue. See also George Mann Burrows, *Commentaries on the Causes, Forms, Symptoms, and Treatment, Moral and Medical, of Insanity* (London, 1828), 109–10, 116, 128–29, 131.

### Chapter 3: The Development of a Medical Jurisprudence of Insanity

1. See the Commission on Lunacy [Levi Lincoln, Edward Jarvis, and Increase Sumner], *Report on Insanity and Idiocy in Massachusetts* (Boston, 1855). Henry M. Hurd, ed., *History of the Institutional Care of the Insane in the United States and Canada* (Baltimore, 1916), 1, 16. For the circumstances surrounding the establishment of the Association, see Hurd, 1, 11–16. See also Deutsch, *The Mentally Ill in America*, 1949 ed., 194–212; Grob, *Mental Institutions in America*, 132–73; and John Albert Pitts, "The Association of Medical Superintendents of American Institutions for the Insane, 1844–1892: A Case Study of Specialism in American Medicine," Ph.D. dissertation, University of Pennsylvania, 1978. Throughout the remainder of this study, the Association of Medical Superintendents of American Institutions for the Insane, the American Medico-Psychological Association, and the American Psychiatric Association will be referred to as "the Association." For an analysis of the difficulties surrounding acceptance of the reality that insanity was not so easily cured, see Deutsch, *The Mentally Ill in America*, 1949 ed., 132–57. See also Dain, *Concepts of Insanity*, 115–17, 125–30.
2. Thomas Story Kirkbride, *On the Construction, Organization, and General Arrangements of Hospitals for the Insane* (Philadelphia, 1854). See also Nancy J. Tomes, *The Persuasive Institution: Thomas Story Kirkbride and the Art of Asylum Keeping* (New York, 1984). Tomes suggests that Kirkbride projected a therapeutic image of the asylum that was designed to obtain middle-class patronage.
3. Annual Report, The Asylum for the Relief of Persons Deprived of the Use of Their Reason, Frankfort, Pennsylvania, 1851–1870. See also annual reports of the following institutions: Boston Lunatic Asylum, 1840–54; Connecticut Retreat for the Insane, 1826 through 1869–70; Eastern Lunatic Asylum, 1868–70; Maine Insane Hospital, 1840–70; Massachusetts General Hospital, McLean Asylum, 1823–70; Mount Hope Hospital, 1842–70 [Mount St. Vincent's Hospital, 1842]; New Hampshire Asylum for the Insane, 1842–70; New York State Lunatic Asylum, 1844–70; Ohio Lunatic Asylum, 1854–70; Government Hospital for the Insane, 1855–70; West Virginia Hospital for the Insane, 1864–70; and the Western Lunatic Asylum, 1851–70.
4. Smith, *Trial by Medicine*, 34–40. See also Thomas C. Upham, *Abridgement of Mental Philosophy* (Boston, 1861), especially the section on the propensities, 336; Waldinger, "Sleep of Reason: John P. Gray and the Challenge of Moral Insanity," 163–79; S. P. Fullinwider, "Insanity or the Loss of Self: The Moral

Insanity Controversy Revisited," *Bulletin of the History of Medicine*, 49 (1975), 87–101; and Dain, *Concepts of Insanity*, 61–62.

5. Winslow, "On Medico-Legal Evidence in Cases of Insanity," *American Journal of Insanity*, 9 (1853), 374.

6. Winslow, *The Plea of Insanity in Criminal Cases* (London, 1843), 53. See also Winslow, "On Medico-Legal Evidence in Cases of Insanity," 375–76; Winslow, "The Legal Doctrine of Responsibility in Cases of Insanity, Connection with Alleged Criminal Acts," *American Journal of Insanity*, 15 (1858), 156–94; and Smith, *Trial by Medicine*, 37.

7. Taylor, *A Manual of Medical Jurisprudence* (London, 1844), 504.

8. [Theodric Romeyn Beck], review of the Taylor work, *American Journal of Insanity*, 2 (1845), 85–86.

9. Taylor, *A Manual of Medical Jurisprudence*, 506.

10. [Brigham], "Danger of Permitting the Insane to Have Their Liberty," *American Journal of Insanity*, 4 (1848), 369–70. See also "Report of the Trustees, Steward, and Superintendent of the Insane Hospital of Augusta, Maine, 1853, Augusta, 1854," *American Journal of Insanity*, 11 (1855), 271. In this annual report, Brigham reported a case of judicial removal with tragic result: "Michael Ward, of Whitefield, in a fit of insanity struck his brother with an axe, and deprived him for life of the use of one of his arms. He was, thereupon, sent to the hospital. Soon after the passing of the act of August, 1849, the selectmen of Whitefield took Ward from the hospital, though warned by the superintendent of his dangerous character, and that insane persons with a homicidal tendency could never be trusted, as they had been known to commit murders after long periods of apparent saneness and quietness. Upon the principle of economy, Ward was set up at auction by the selectmen of Whitefield, to be kept by the lowest bidder. Michael Skane, a friend and countryman, fearing that he would not be properly taken care of by the person to whom he was knocked off, after consulting his wife, was led, by a feeling of compassion for a fellow-countryman, to take him at the low price for which he was bid off. His humanity cost him his life. Ward, in a fit of frenzy, killed his friend who had been taking care of him, and then absconded. He had been very recently captured, and is now in Wiscasset jail, awaiting to take his trial at the supreme court. The trustees would, therefore, most earnestly urge the repeal of the law of August 14, 1849."

11. William H. Stokes, "The Eleventh Annual Report of the Mount Hope Institution, near Baltimore, Maryland, for the Year 1853," *American Journal of Insanity*, 11 (1855), 263. See also John Minson Galt, "On the Medico-Legal Question of the Confinement of the Insane," *American Journal of Insanity*, 9 (1853), 217–23; "Insanity and Crime," *American Journal of Insanity*, 14 (1858), 404; "Proceedings of the Association," *American Journal of Insanity*, 23 (1866), 90; and "Reports of Lunatic Asylums," *American Journal of Insanity*, 25 (1869), 368. For a discussion of the overcrowding of asylums, see Dain, *Concepts of Insanity*, 128–33. See also Grob, *Mental Institutions in America*, 257–69.

12. [Brigham], "Authority to Restrain the Insane, Supreme Judicial Court of Massachusetts, January 1845, at Boston: Matter of Josiah Oakes," *American Journal of Insanity*, 2 (1846), 224–34. The Josiah Oakes decision established the right of the state to restrain the insane solely on the basis of "aberration

of mind." For a discussion of the most notable of these incidents, see Grob, *Mental Institutions in America*, 63–69. See also "Reports of Hospitals for the Insane," *American Journal of Insanity*, 8 (1851), 174–75; Isaac Ray, *A Treatise on the Medical Jurisprudence of Insanity*, 4th ed. (Boston, 1860), 369; and William H. Stokes, "Mount Hope Institution—Trial for Conspiracy," *American Journal of Insanity*, 23 (1866), 311–29.

13. "Summary, Murders by the Insane," *American Journal of Insanity*, 20 (1863), 246.

14. Ray, "Project of a Law Determining the Legal Relations of the Insane," *American Journal of Insanity*, 7 (1851), 215–34; Ray, "American Legislation on Insanity," *American Journal of Insanity*, 21 (1864), 21–62. See also Dr. Parigot, "The Social Relations of the Insane in Civil and Criminal Cases," *American Journal of Insanity*, 21 (1865), 477–96. For a comprehensive treatment of the history of the legal aspects of psychiatry, see Hurd, *The Institutional Care of the Insane*, 1, 321–37; and Deutsch, *The Mentally Ill in America*, 1949 ed., 418–41.

15. Dain, *Concepts of Insanity*, 82–83.

16. [Gray], "Trial of Robert C. Sloo for the Murder of John E. Hall—Defense: Insanity," *American Journal of Insanity*, 15 (1858), 33–68. See also Waldinger, "Sleep of Reason: John P. Gray and the Challenge of Moral Insanity," 163–79.

17. [Gray], "Case of Elizabeth Heggie," *American Journal of Insanity*, 25 (1868), 20. Cook was Superintendent of Brigham Hall, Canandaigua, New York; Brown was Superintendent of Bloomingdale Asylum, New York City.

18. Gray, "Homicide in Insanity," *American Journal of Insanity*, 14 (1857), 143.

19. *Ibid.*, 142. See also [Gray], "Moral Insanity," *American Journal of Insanity*, 14 (1858), 311–22; [Gray], "The Case of William Speirs—Arson: Plea of Insanity," *American Journal of Insanity*, 15 (1858), 200–25; Ray, "An Examination of the Objections to the Doctrine of Moral Insanity," *American Journal of Insanity*, 18 (1861), 112–38; and [Gray], "Dr. Ray on Moral Insanity," *American Journal of Insanity*, 18 (1861), 83–88.

20. Bucknill and Tuke, *A Manual of Psychological Medicine* (London, 1858).

21. *Ibid.*, 322.

22. *Ibid.*, 324.

## Chapter 4: From Static Brain to Dynamic Neurophysiology, 1840–1870

1. [Brigham], "Cases Illustrative of the Medical Jurisprudence of Insanity," *American Journal of Insanity*, 1 (1844), 67.

2. "Reports of American Asylums," *American Journal of Insanity*, 21 (1864), 246.

3. "Proceedings of the Association," *American Journal of Insanity*, 20 (1863), 76–79.

4. For a discussion of Griesinger, see Menninger, *The Vital Balance*, 454. See also Klaus Doerner, *Madmen and the Bourgeoisie*, trans. Joachim Neugroschel and Jean Steinberg (Oxford, 1981), 270–90.

5. Ordronaux, "History and Philosophy of Medical Jurisprudence," *American Journal of Insanity*, 25 (1868), 205. See also Norman Dain and Eric T. Carlson,

"Moral Insanity in the United States, 1835–1866," *American Journal of Psychiatry*, 118 (1962), 797–98.

6. Chipley, "In Court of Appeals, State of Kentucky, Smith vs. Commonwealth with Remarks," *American Journal of Insanity*, 23 (1866), 29–32.

7. "Proceedings of the Association," *American Journal of Insanity*, 23 (1866), 93–96.

8. Dain, *Concepts of Insanity*, 79.

9. Ray, *Medical Jurisprudence*, 1838 ed., 232–33.

10. C. Lockhard-Robertson and Henry Maudsley, *Insanity and Crime: Medico-Legal Commentary on the Case of George Victor Townley* (London, 1864), 15. For Gray's review of this case, see "Summary," *American Journal of Insanity*, 19 (1862), 243–46. See also [Gray], "Moral Insanity," *American Journal of Insanity*, 22 (1865), 133–37.

11. Lockhard-Robertson and Maudsley, *Insanity and Crime*, 9.

12. *Ibid.*, 23.

13. *Ibid.*, 30–33.

14. Prichard, *On the Different Forms of Insanity*, 130.

15. Bucknill and Tuke, *A Manual of Psychological Medicine*, 1858 ed., 201. By this time, most alienists used the term "irresistible impulse" to designate a paroxysm of violence motivated by delusion or hallucination.

16. Woodward, "Homicidal Impulse," *American Journal of Insanity*, 1 (1845), 324.

17. Maudsley, "Homicidal Insanity," *Journal of Mental Science*, 9 (1863), 327–43. See also C. Lockhard-Robertson, "A Case of Homicidal Mania without Disorder of the Intellect," *Journal of Mental Science*, 6 (1859–60), 386–98; Edward Jarvis, "Mania Transitoria," *American Journal of Insanity*, 26 (1869), 1–32. After reviewing the literature and the reported cases in this paper, Jarvis concluded that, if such a condition existed, it was indeed rare.

18. [Gray], "The Case of David M. Wright for the Murder of Lieutenant Sandborn—Plea: Insanity," *American Journal of Insanity*, 20 (1864), 284.

19. *Ibid.*, 299.

20. Ray, "The Case of Bernard Clangley," *American Journal of Insanity*, 22 (1865), 25–26.

21. *Ibid.*, 31.

22. "Proceedings of the Association," *American Journal of Insanity*, 22 (1865), 44.

23. *Ibid.*, 39. Gray was not present at the discussion.

24. Burrows, *Commentaries*, 156.

25. Maudsley, *The Physiology and Pathology of Mind*, 2nd ed. (London, 1868), 402. See also Jules Falret, "On Moral Insanity," *American Journal of Insanity*, 23 (1867), 546.

26. "Reports of American Asylums," *American Journal of Insanity*, 21 (1864), 245. See also "On the Action of Bromide of Potassium," *American Journal of Insanity*, 21 (1864), 301–03; "Proceedings of the Association," *American Journal of Insanity*, 22 (1865), 64–65; "Reports of American Hospitals for the Insane for 1867," *American Journal of Insanity*, 24 (1868), 424; and "Bromide of Potassium in Epilepsy," *American Journal of Insanity*, 24 (1864), 494. For a more detailed account of the medical treatment of epilepsy, see J. Russell Reynolds, *Epilepsy: Its Symptoms, Treatment, and Relation to Other Chronic, Convulsive Diseases* (London, 1861).

27. Ray, "Epilepsy and Homicide," *American Journal of Insanity*, 24 (1867), 190.
28. *Ibid.*, 196.
29. See especially Henri F. Ellenberger, *The Discovery of the Unconscious: The History and Evolution of Dynamic Psychiatry* (New York, 1970), 284–85. See also S. P. Fullinwider, *Technicians of the Finite: The Rise and Decline of the Schizophrenic in American Thought, 1840–1960* (Westport, Connecticut, 1982), 31, 59.
30. See, for example, Charles P. Bancroft, "Subconscious Homicide and Suicide: Their Physiological Psychology," *American Journal of Insanity*, 55 (1898), 263–73.
31. Maudsley, *The Physiology and Pathology of Mind*, 1868 ed., 1–2.
32. For Maudsley's influence as a jurisprudent, see Smith, *Trial by Medicine*. 13, 25, 51–57.
33. Maudsley, *The Physiology and Pathology of Mind*, 1868 ed., 42–44, 362. Gray disagreed with Maudsley on the question of whether the moral sense could be left unaffected by neurophysiology. See Gray's review of the Maudsley work, *American Journal of Insanity*, 24 (1868), 336–60.
34. Maudsley, *The Physiology and Pathology of Mind*, 1868 ed., 372.

## Chapter 5: The Non-Asylum Treatment of the Insane

1. Erwin A. Ackernecht, *A Short History of Psychiatry*, trans. Sulammith Wolfe (New York, 1959), 47–51. See also Arthur E. Fink, *Causes of Crime: Biological Theories in the United States, 1880–1915* (Philadelphia, 1938); Mark H. Haller, *Eugenics: Hereditarian Attitudes in American Thought, 1870–1930* (New Brunswick, New Jersey, 1963); Charles Rosenberg, "Charles Benedict Davenport and the Beginning of Human Genetics," *Bulletin of the History of Medicine*, 35 (1961), 266–76; Charles H. Hughes, "History of the O.Z. Family: An Illustration of Rapid Neuropathic Degeneracy," *Alienist and Neurologist*, 3 (1882), 535–38; Hughes, "The Rights of the Insane," *Alienist and Neurologist*, 4 (1883), 183–89.
2. For a summary of the development of neurology and its impact upon psychiatry, see Deutsch, *The Mentally Ill in America*, 1949 ed., 276–83; Jacques M. Quen, "Asylum Psychiatry, Neurology, Social Work, and Mental Hygiene: An Exploratory Study in Interprofessional History," *Journal of the History of the Behavioral Sciences*, 13 (1977), 3–11; and Bonnie Ellen Blustein, "A Hollow Square of Psychological Science: American Neurologists and Psychiatrists in Conflict," in Scull, *Madness*, 241–70.
3. Hurd, *History*, 331–43. See also Deutsch, *The Mentally Ill in America* 1949 ed., 418–41; "Code of Law Relating to the Insane in New York, Passed May 1874," *American Journal of Insanity*, 31 (1874), 80–89; "Revision of the New York Lunacy Code," *American Journal of Insanity*, 39 (1881), 116–17; "Lunacy Law in Illinois," *American Journal of Insanity*, 47 (1891), 584–87; Stephen Smith, "Unification of Laws of the States Relating to the Commitment of the Insane," *American Journal of Insanity*, 49 (1892), 157–83; and George L. Harrison, *Legislation on Insanity* (New York, 1884).
4. A. E. MacDonald, "The Examination and Commitment of the Insane," *American Journal of Insanity*, 32 (1876), 505.

5. *Ibid.*
6. Fox, *So Far Disordered in Mind: Insanity in California, 1870–1930* (Berkeley, 1978), 38–40.
7. Gray, "English Lunacy Law," *American Journal of Insanity* (1880), 460. See also Bucknill, *The Care of the Insane and Their Legal Control*, 2nd ed. (London, 1880), 46. Bucknill concludes: "The sole purpose of the law is to provide for the safety of the public and the individual. Safety is the one sole object which the law of England recognizes as the aim and purpose of confining the insane. Where there is no danger, there can be no legal justification of confinement; and, without doubt, any harmless and safe person, however insane, would be entitled to damages for confinement in an asylum, even if by such confinement he had received the greatest medical benefit in regard of his disease."
8. Bucknill, *The Care of the Insane*, 2nd ed., 46. See also John Ordronaux, *Judicial Aspects of Insanity* (Albany, New York, 1878).
9. Foster Pratt, "Insane Patients and Their Legal Relations," *American Journal of Insanity*, 35 (1878), 182.
10. Hammond, *The Non-Asylum Treatment of the Insane* (New York, 1879), 2.
11. Stephen Smith, "Remarks on the Lunacy Laws of the State of New York as Regards the Provisions for Commitment and Discharge of the Insane," *American Journal of Insanity*, 40 (1883), 50–70. See also "Report on the Lunacy Laws of the State of New York," *American Journal of Insanity*, 40 (1883), 102–09.
12. Smith, *The Commitment and Detention of the Insane in the United States: Report of a Committee to the National Conference of Charities in Buffalo, [New York], June 7, 1888* (Boston, 1888). The members of the committee were: Smith, chairman, New York City; Fred H. Wines, Springfield, Illinois; A. O. Wright, Madison, Wisconsin; Henry M. Hoyt, Philadelphia, Pennsylvania; Richard Gundry, M.D., Catonsville, Maryland; F. B. Sanborn, Concord, Massachusetts.
13. Fox, *So Far Disordered in Mind*, 36, 75. Fox pointed this irony out in connection with the sterilization campaign in California between 1890 and 1920. Alienists tended to commit lunatics with the assumption that they would be rendered harmless before they were discharged.
14. Hurd, "Recent Judicial Decisions in Michigan Relative to Insanity," *American Journal of Insanity*, 37 (1880), 28.
15. *Ibid.*, 33.
16. "Proceedings of the Association of Medical Superintendents," *American Journal of Insanity*, 33 (1976), 309. See also Jamin Strong, "Twenty-seventh Annual Report of the Cleveland Asylum for the Insane," *American Journal of Insanity*, 39 (1883), 483–86; John P. Gray, "Judge Lawrence and the Release of Lunatics," *American Journal of Insanity*, 40 (1884), 521; "Lord Chief Justice Cockburn on the Responsibility of the Insane," *American Journal of Insanity*, 38 (1881), 60–72; Bucknill, "A Lecture on the Relation of Madness to Crime," *American Journal of Insanity*, 40 (1884), 412–39; and Gray, "English Lunacy Law," 463.
17. See for example, Henry M. Hurd, "The Data of Recovery from Insanity," *American Journal of Insanity*, 43 (1886), 243–55; and "Proceedings of the Association of Medical Superintendents," *American Journal of Insanity*, 32 (1876), 334.
18. "Proceedings of the Association," 338.

19. *Ibid.*, 341.
20. "Proceedings of the Association," *American Journal of Insanity*, 33 (1876), 183–85.
21. Landor, "Probationary Leaves of Absence," *American Journal of Insanity*, 32 (1876), 481.
22. "Proceedings of the Association," 295–99.
23. *Ibid.*, 310. However, MacDonald equivocates on this issue in a paper in the same volume; see his "Examination and Commitment of the Insane," 505.
24. "Proceedings of the Association," 296–97.
25. Hurd, *History*, 1, 258–80. See also H. M. Bannister, "The Home Treatment of Insanity," *Journal of Nervous and Mental Disease*, 22 (1895), 718–28; and Adolf Meyer, "Reception Hospitals, Psychopathic Wards, and Psychopathic Hospitals," *American Journal of Insanity*, 64 (1907), 221–30; Fox, *So Far Disordered in Mind*, 58–59.
26. Owen Copp, "Further Experience in Family Care of the Insane in Massachusetts," *American Journal of Insanity*, 63 (1907), 361–75.
27. *Ibid.*, 372.

## Chapter 6: Homicidal Insanity and the Unstable Nervous System, 1870–1910

1. For a summary of the changes in somatic theories of insanity from 1850 to 1879 in Great Britain and their relationships to the practice of physicians, see L. S. Jacyna, "Somatic Theories of Mind and the Interests of Medicine in Britain," *Medical History*, 26 (1982), 259–78. See also A. E. MacDonald, "The Examination and Commitment of the Insane," *American Journal of Insanity*, 32 (1876), 515; and Allan McLane Hamilton, "The Development of the Legal Relations Concerning the Insane, with Suggestions for Reform," *Medical Record*, 74 (1908), 781–88.
2. Isaac Ray, *A Treatise on the Medical Jurisprudence of Insanity*, 5th ed. (Boston, 1871), 26–27. See also Henry Maudsley, *Responsibility in Mental Disease* (London, 1874), 77–80, 99, 128; Edward C. Mann, *Insanity: Its Etiology, Diagnosis, Pathology, and Treatment, with Cases Illustrating Pathology, Morbid Histology, and Treatment* (New York, 1875), 4; John Charles Bucknill and Daniel Hack Tuke, *A Manual of Psychological Medicine*, 4th ed. (London, 1879) 50, 269; Hammond, *A Treatise on Insanity in Its Medical Relations*, 273; and Spitzka, *Insanity*, 24, 286–93.
3. Menninger, *The Vital Balance*, 457–64 (Menninger traces the evolution of Kraepelin's nosology throughout the nine editions of the textbook); William D. Granger, "Monomania," *American Journal of Insanity*, 41 (1885), 416–17. See also William McDonald, "The Present Status of Paranoia," *American Journal of Insanity*, 60 (1904), 476; G. W. Page, "Paranoid Dementia," *American Journal of Insanity*, 60 (1904), 525–35; Walter Channing, "The Evolution of Paranoia: Report of a Case," *Journal of Nervous and Mental Disease*, 19 (1892), 142–214; Edward N. Flint, "A Case of Paranoia," *Journal of Nervous and Mental Disease*, 20 (1898), 567–78; Robert H. Chase. "Delusions of the Insane," *Journal of Nervous and Mental Disease*, 32 (1905), 454–63; and M. S. Gregory, "Dis-

cussion of the Present-Day Limitation of the Conception of Paranoia," *Journal of Nervous and Mental Disease*, 35 (1908), 656–60.

4. Maudsley, *Responsibility in Mental Disease*, 224. See also Bucknill and Tuke *A Manual of Psychological Medicine*, 1879 ed., 224–25; Mann, *Insanity*, 12–13; Spitzka, *Insanity*, 313; Thomas S. Clouston, *Clinical Lectures on Mental Disease* (London, 1883), 105; G. Fielding Blandford, *Insanity and Its Treatment*, 3rd ed. (New York, 1886), 129; Theodore Kirchoff, *Handbook of Insanity for Practitioners and Students* (New York, 1893), 254; Theodore H. Kellogg, *A Text-Book of Mental Diseases* (New York, 1897), 387–88; Archibald Church and Frederick Peterson, *Nervous and Mental Diseases*, 3rd ed. (Philadelphia, 1901), 691; A Ross Defendorf [Diefendorf], *Clinical Psychiatry: A Text-Book for Students and Physicians, Abstracted and Adapted from the Sixth German Edition of Kraepelin's "Lehrbuch der Psychiatrie,"* (New York, 1902), 69, 324; R. von Krafft-Ebing, *Text-Book of Insanity*, trans. Charles Gilbert Chaddock (Philadelphia, 1905), 385; and William A. White, *Outlines of Psychiatry* (New York, 1908), 100.

5. Folsom, "Case of Charles F. Freeman of Pocasset, Massachusetts—Tried for Murder of His Child—Sentenced for Life to the Massachusetts State Hospital, Danvers," *American Journal of Insanity*, 40 (1884), 362.

6. Charles E. Rosenberg, *The Trial of the Assassin Guiteau*, (Chicago, 1968), especially Spitzka's testimony, 155–77. See also Spitzka, *Insanity*, 294–95; Addison S. Thayer, "Five Maine Murders," *Boston Medical Surgical Journal*, 146 (1902), 215–19; Edward C. Mann, "The Trial of Dr. L. U. Beach, of Pennsylvania, with His Psychological and Pathological History," *Alienist and Neurologist*, 6 (1885), 325–33; and Walter Channing, "The Mental Status of Czolgosz, the Assassin of President McKinley," *American Journal of Insanity*, 59 (1902), 233–78.

7. Hammond, *Insanity in Its Relation to Crime* (New York, 1873), 48, 60–61.

8. William Wilkins Carr, "The Webber Murder Case in Philadelphia," *Medico-Legal Journal*, 6 (1888–89), 243–62.

9. Carlson and Dain, "The Meaning of Moral Insanity," 130–40.

10. "Proceedings of the Association of Medical Superintendents," *American Journal of Insanity*, 29 (1872), 155. See also John Ordronaux, "Moral Insanity," *American Journal of Insanity*, 29 (1873), 313–40; Rosenberg, *The Trial of the Assassin Guiteau*, 163–64; Spitzka, *Insanity*, 56; John P. Gray, "Ulterior Consideration on the Discussion of the So-Called Moral Insanity," *American Journal of Insanity*, 36 (1879), 224–29; Joseph Workman, "Bonfigli on Moral Insanity," *American Journal of Insanity*, 36 (1880), 476–96; and Joseph Workman, "Moral Insanity—What Is It?" *American Journal of Insanity*, 39 (1883), 334–48.

11. H. H. Bannister, "Moral Insanity," *Journal of Nervous and Mental Disease*, 4 (1877), 645–48. See also Hammond, *A Treatise on Insanity*, 432.

12. See, for example, W. Bevan-Lewis, *A Text-Book of Mental Diseases*, 2nd ed. (London, 1899), 394–95; Defendorf [Diefendorf], *Clinical Psychiatry*, 403–04; C. H. Hughes, "Imbecility and the Insanity of Imbecility before the Law. Murder by Suggestion. The State of Missouri vs. Benj. Cronenbold, Charged with Murder in the First Degree. A Medico-Legal Record," *Alienist and Neurologist*, 20 (1899), 187–215; Edward C. Mann, "The Legal Relations of

Imbecility and of Suicidal and Homicidal Mania," *Brooklyn Medical Journal*, 4 (1890), 132–39; and P. Bryce, "Biennial Reports of the Alabama Insane Hospital, Tuscaloosa, Ala., for the Years Ending September 30, 1885 and 1886," *American Journal of Insanity*, 43 (1887), 372.

13. Spitzka, *Insanity*, 281.
14. C. K. Clarke, "The Case of William B.: Moral Imbecility," *American Journal of Insanity*, 43 (1886), 83–103.
15. *Ibid.*, 89.
16. Henry R. Stedman, "A Case of Moral Insanity with Repeated Homicides and Incendiarism and Late Development of Delusions," *American Journal of Insanity*, 61 (1904), 284–85; Menninger, *The Vital Balance*, 458–59; Defendorf [Diefendorf], *Clinical Psychiatry*, 403–04. See also Kraepelin, *Lectures on Clinical Psychiatry. Edited and Revised by Thomas Johnstone* (London, 1904), 285–92.
17. White, *Outlines of Psychiatry*, 1908 ed., 219–20.
18. Gray, "Responsibility of the Insane: Homicide in Insanity," 13. See also "Proceedings of the Association of Medical Superintendents," 32 (1876), 362; Ordronaux, "Moral Insanity," 331.
19. Spitzka, *Insanity*, 36–37.
20. Ray, *Treatise on the Medical Jurisprudence of Insanity*, 1871 ed., 222; Maudsley, *Responsibility in Mental Disease*, 150–73; Bucknill and Tuke, *A Manual of Psychological Medicine*, 1879 ed., 255, 257; Hammond, *A Treatise on Insanity*, 389–91; Spitzka, *Insanity*, 35–38; Clouston, *Clinical Lectures on Mental Disease*, 244–47; Blandford, *Insanity and Its Treatment*, 131, 239; Daniel Hack Tuke, ed., *Dictionary of Psychological Medicine* (London, 1892), 1, 593–94; Kellogg, *A Text Book of Mental Diseases*, 750–51; Defendorf [Diefendorf], *Clinical Psychiatry*, 389–91; Charles L. Dana, *A Textbook of Nervous Diseases and Psychiatry*, 6th ed. (New York, 1904), 632–33; Bevan-Lewis, *A Text Book of Mental Diseases*, 108–16; White, *Outlines of Psychiatry*, 1908 ed., 58.
21. Prince, "A Case of 'Imperative Idea' or 'Homicidal Impulse' in a Neurasthenic without Hereditary Taint," *Boston Medical and Surgical Journal*, 136 (1897), 57. See also George M. Beard, *A Practical Treatise on Nervous Exhaustion (Neurasthenia): Its Symptoms, Nature, Sequences, Treatment* (New York, 1880).
22. Wigglesworth, "Case of Murder, the Result of Pure Homicidal Impulse," *Journal of Mental Science*, 47 (1901), 338.
23. Menninger, *The Vital Balance*, 458–59. See also Defendorf, *Clinical Psychiatry*, 1912 ed., 226–27.
24. Hitchcock, "A Case of Dementia Praecox of Medico-Legal Interest," *American Journal of Insanity*, 62 (1906), 623.
25. Ray, *Treatise on the Medical Jurisprudence of Insanity*, 5th ed. (Boston, 1871), 149–50.
26. Spitzka, *Insanity*, 154.
27. Hammond, *A Treatise on Insanity*, 522; Clouston, *Clinical Lectures on Mental Diseases*, 1884 ed., 161; Spitzka, *Insanity*, 155. See also Evan Powell, "Unconscious Homicidal and Suicidal Impulse," *Journal of Mental Science*, 32 (1886–87), 500–03; and P. Bryce, "A Case of Mania Transitoria," *American Journal of Insanity*, 45 (1889), 442–45.
28. Maudsley, *Responsibility in Mental Disease*, 247.
29. *Ibid.*, 247–48. See also Bucknill and Tuke, *A Manual of Psychological Medicine*,

1879 ed., 259; Blandford, *Insanity and Its Treatment*, 155–56; Kellogg, *A Text Book of Mental Diseases*, 725, 729; Bevan-Lewis, *A Text-Book of Mental Diseases*, 215; and W. J. Conklin, *The Relations of Epilepsy to Insanity and Jurisprudence*, Address before the Ohio State Medical Society, April 6, 1871, 43 pp.

30. "Proceedings of the Association of Medical Superintendents," *American Journal of Insanity*, 29 (1872), 142.

31. MacDonald, "Case of Edmund J. Hoppin, Homicide—Plea: Insanity," *American Journal of Insanity*, 34 (1878), 462–511. See also S. T. Clarke, "Case of Pierce, Plea, Insanity: What is Mania Transitoria? Who Are Liable? How Should It Affect Jurisprudence?" *American Journal of Insanity*, 28 (1872), 399–409. Clarke, superintendent of the insane asylum at Canandaigua testified against the existence of *mania transitoria* in this case, but the prisoner was acquitted.

32. John C. Bucknill and Daniel H. Tuke, *A Manual of Psychological Medicine*, 2nd ed. (London, 1862), 283–84. See also Tuke, *Dictionary of Psychological Medicine*, 2, 1302–03 (the article on *mania transitoria* was contributed by Otto von Schwartzer, physician-in-chief, Private Sanatorium for Mental and Nervous Diseases, Budapest); Maudsley, *Responsibility in Mental Disease*, 268–69; E. Mesnet, "The Automatism of Memory and Association in Pathological Somnambulism," *The Chicago Journal of Nervous and Mental Disease*, 2 (1875), 48–67; and Francis H. Wamsley, *Outlines of Insanity* (London, 1892), 28.

33. John P. Gray, "The McFarland Trial," *American Journal of Insanity*, 27 (1881), 265–77.

34. Thomas S. Clouston, "The McFarland Trial," *Journal of Mental Science*, 16 (1870), 421.

35. *Ibid.*, 423–24.

36. See, for example, Spitzka's argument in *Insanity*, 154. See also Tuke, *Dictionary of Psychological Medicine*, 2, 1302; P. Bryce, "A Case of Mania Transitoria," *American Journal of Insanity*, 45 (1889), 442–45; and George Pitt-Lewis, R. Percy Smith, and J. A. Hawke, *The Insane and the Law: A Plain Guide for Medical Men, Solicitors, and Others* (London, 1895), 5.

37. The British physician W. Bevan-Lewis, medical director of the West Riding Asylum, in the second edition (1899) of his textbook, made an observation in this connection:
    "Amongst other etiological factors, we must not fail to note the vicious agency of imitation which was originally emphasized by Esquirol, as one of the causes of this affection. Undoubtedly, the morbid excitement engendered by the perusal of records of criminal horrors, by the publicity afforded in our Assize Courts to the revolting details of crime, and, up to within the last few years, the demoralizing effect of public executions have greatly fostered the development of these states of mental disease. . . . The brutal instincts are still less protected in those persons of weak mind, who, not endowed with an average amount of controlling power, require by the intensification of such instinctive states to lead to explosive outbursts; in such cases mental strain, anxiety, ill-health, and other exhausting conditions, and especially alcoholic and sexual intemperance, may readily lead to attacks of homicidal mania at periods when the public mind is horrified by some startling crime." Bevan-Lewis, *A Text-Book of Mental Disease*, 215–16.

38. Temkin, Oswei, *"The Falling Sickness,"* 2nd ed. (Baltimore, 1971), 308–09. See also Jackson, "On Temporary Mental Disorders after Epileptic Paroxysm," in James Taylor, ed., *Selected Writings of John Hughlings Jackson,* (New York, 1958), 1, 119–34; Jackson, *Clinical and Physiological Researches on the Nervous System* (London, 1875); and Jackson, *Neurological Fragments* (London, 1925).

39. P. M. Wise, "The Barber Case: The Legal Responsibility of Epileptics," *American Journal of Insanity,* 45 (1889), 360–73. See also "Medical Jurisprudence. The People, Resp'ts vs. Richard Barber, App't.," *American Journal of Insanity,* 46 (1890), 375–89; "Automatic Homicide," *The British Medical Journal,* January 2, 1886, 26; and William C. Kraus, "The People vs. Sadie McMullen: A Medico-Legal Case," *Journal of Nervous and Mental Disease,* 18 (1891), 416. See, for example, Henry R. Stedman, "A Case of Insanity Resulting in Homicide and Attempted Family Slaughter and Suicide," *Alienist and Neurologist,* 6 (1886), 99–106; J. K. Baudy, "Epilepsy in its Medico-Legal Relations to the Case of Max Klingler," *St. Louis Medical and Surgical Journal* (1870), 507; and William A. Hammond, *A Treatise on the Diseases of the Nervous System,* 6th ed. (New York, 1876), 675. Hammond believed that the epileptic's crimes were excusable if they were directly connected with the paroxysm.

40. Manuel Gonzalez Echeverria, *On Epilepsy: Anatomo-Pathological and Clinical Notes* (New York, 1870), 368. See also Maudsley, *Responsibility in Mental Disease,* 245, 248; Bucknill and Tuke, *A Manual of Psychological Medicine,* 1879 ed., 336–44; W. R. Gowers, *Epilepsy and Other Chronic Convulsive Diseases: Their Causes, Symptoms, and Treatment* (New York, 1885), 95–96; Hammond, *A Treatise on Insanity,* 639; Spitzka, *Insanity,* 261, 265–67; Clouston, *Clinical Lectures,* 287, 294; Blandford, *Insanity and Its Treatment,* 60–61, 130; Tuke, *A Dictionary of Psychological Medicine,* 1, 453–54; W. R. Gowers, *A Manual of Diseases of the Nervous System* (Philadelphia, 1893), 2, 748; Bevan-Lewis, *A Text-Book of Mental Diseases,* 260–61, 268–69, 274; Church and Peterson, *Nervous and Mental Diseases,* 1901 ed., 742–43; Defendorf [Diefendorf], *Clinical Psychiatry,* 1902 ed., 336, 338–39; William P. Spratling, *Epilepsy and Its Treatment* (Philadelphia, 1904), 446–49; and A. O. Kellogg, "Epilepsy and Its Relations to Insanity—and Cases of Doubtful Responsiblility before Judicial Tribunals, with Remarks on Expert Testimony," *Quarterly Journal of Psychological Medicine and Medical Jurisprudence,* 6 (1872), 660–61.

41. John Ordronaux, "Case of Isabella Jenisch: Epileptic Homicide," *American Journal of Insanity,* 31 (1875), 431.

42. Gowers, *Epilepsy,* 96. See also Tuke, *Dictionary of Psychological Medicine,* 1, 451, 453.

43. Echeverria, *On Epilepsy,* 362, 267–68. See also Maudsley, *Responsibility in Mental Disease,* 96–102; and "Special Provision for Epileptics," *American Journal of Insanity,* 48 (1892), 409–10.

44. Echeverria, *On Epilepsy,* 363; Maudsley, *Responsibility in Mental Disease,* 250; Gowers, *Epilepsy,* 101–02; Spitzka, *Insanity,* 261; Clouston, *Clinical Lectures,* 1883 ed., 287–88, 294; Tuke, *Dictionary of Psychological Medicine,* 1, 455; Kellogg, *A Text Book of Mental Disease,* 577–81; Bevan-Lewis, *A Text-Book of Mental Diseases,* 274–75, 277; Church and Peterson, *Nervous and Mental Diseases,* 1901 ed., 747; Defendorf [Diefendorf], *Clinical Psychiatry,* 1902 ed., 336–

38; Clouston, *Clinical Lectures*, 1904 ed., 442; Spratling, *Epilepsy and Its Treatment*, 449–50; Kraepelin, *Lectures on Clinical Psychiatry*, 52.
45. John Ordronaux, "Case of Jacob Staudermann," *American Journal of Insanity*, 32 (1876), 453. Ordronaux regarded Staudermann, an epileptic who committed a homicide, as "one member of this broken down class of human beings." By this designation, Ordronaux meant immigrants, who in his opinion should not be admitted into the country because of their degeneracy. Like many, if not most of his contemporaries, he was opposed to free immigration. He believed that "America is becoming, in fact, a sort of international dust bin, into which, the old civilizations sweep their human refuse." 456. See also Echeverria, *On Epilepsy*, 362; Conklin, *The Relations of Epilepsy to Insanity*, 20; C. Adler Blumner, "A Case of Perverted Sexual Instinct," *American Journal of Insanity*, 39 (1882), 34; John Hughlings Jackson, "On Temporary Mental Disorders after Epileptic Paroxysms," in James Taylor, ed., *Selected Writings of John Hughlings Jackson* (New York, 1958), 1, 128; and "Proceedings of the Association of Medical Superintendents," *American Journal of Insanity*, 36 (1879), 201.
46. Echeverria, *On Epilepsy*, 363.
47. Hurd, *History*, 3, 352, 252–56.
48. Annual Report, Ohio Hospital for Epileptics, Gallipolis, Ohio, 1894. See also State of New York, *Annual Report of the State Board of Charities, Craig Colony for Epileptics*, 1894–1910.
49. Biennial Report, Ohio Hospital for Epileptics, 1908–09, 28.
50. State of New York, *Annual Report of the State Board of Charities, Craig Colony for Epileptics*, 1894–1910.
51. Gray, "Responsibility of the Insane: Homicide in Insanity," *American Journal of Insanity*, 31 (1875) 157.
52. Baker, "Female Criminal Lunatics: A Sketch," *Journal of Mental Science*, 48 (1902), 14, 16.

## Chapter 7: Psychoanalysis and Medical Criminology

1. See especially John C. Burnham, *Psychoanalysis and American Medicine, 1894–1918: Medicine, Science, and Culture* (New York, 1967), 8.
2. Bell, *Treating the Mentally Ill*, 135–63.
3. *Ibid.*, 51. See also, Burnham, "Psychiatry, Psychology, and the Progressive Movement," *American Quarterly*, 12 (1960), 457–65; and Barbara Sicherman, *The Quest for Mental Health in America, 1880–1917* (New York, 1979).
4. Walter Bromberg, *Psychiatry between the Wars, 1918–1945: A Recollection*, (Westport, Connecticut, 1982).
5. Burnham, *Psychoanalysis and American Medicine*. See also Jacques M. Quen and Eric T. Carlson, eds., *American Psychoanalysis: Origins and Development* (New York, 1978); Clarence Oberndorf, *The History of Psychoanalysis in America* (New York, 1953); and Nathan G. Hale, Jr., *Freud and the Americans: The Beginning of Psychoanalysis in the United States, 1876–1917* (New York, 1971).
6. Meyer, "A Science of Man," in Alfred Lief, ed., *The Commonsense Psychiatry*

*of Dr. Adolf Meyer*, (New York, 1948), 537. See also Jacques M. Quen, "Asylum Psychiatry, Neurology, Social Work, and Mental Hygiene," 7.

7. Menninger, *The Vital Balance*, 467.
8. A. A. Brill, "Psychological Mechanisms of Paranoia," *New York Medical Journal*, 94 (1911), 957–74. See also Brill, "Homoerotism and Paranoia," *American Journal of Psychiatry*, 90 (1934), 957–74.
9. Zilboorg, "Dynamics of Schizophrenic Reactions Related to Pregnancy and Childbirth," *American Journal of Psychiatry*, 8 (1929), 733–67. See also Zilboorg, "Depressive Reactions Related to Parenthood," *American Journal of Psychiatry*, 10 (1931), 927–62; and Zilboorg, "Sidelights on Parent-Child Antagonism," *American Journal of Orthopsychiatry*, 2 (1932), 35–43.
10. Bender, "Psychiatric Mechanism in Child Murderers," *Journal of Nervous and Mental Disease*, 80 (1934), 46.
11. L. Pierce Clark, "Further Contribution to the Psychology of the Essential Epileptic," *Journal of Nervous and Mental Disease*, 63 (1926), 575–85; J. Notkin, "Personality Make-up of Epileptics," *Journal of Nervous and Mental Disease*, 65 (1927), 617; L. Pierce Clark, *Epilepsy and the Convulsive State* (Baltimore, 1931), 74.
12. Ellenberger, *The Discovery of the Unconscious*, 803. See also Quen, "Asylum Psychiatry, Neurology, Social Work, and Mental Hygiene," 11.
13. Deutsch, *The Mentally Ill in America*, 442–82, especially pp. 445–46. See also Bell, *Treating the Mentally Ill*, 80–81. Nurse training programs began in 1882 with the program set up by Edward Cowles at the McLean Asylum. By 1893 the Association had appointed a nursing committee. By 1900 there were fifty such schools. See "Proceedings of the Association," *American Journal of Insanity*, 43 (1886), 158–78. These training schools, however, had relatively little impact upon the care of the insane. See John Maurice Grimes, *Institutional Care of Mental Patients in the United States* (Chicago, 1934), 30–31.
14. White, "Scheme for a Standard Minimum Examination of Mental Cases for the Use in Hospitals for the Insane," *American Journal of Insanity*, 67 (1910), 17–24. See also Shepherd Ivory Franz, *Handbook of Mental Examination Methods* (New York, 1912). For comparison, see Bucknill and Tuke, *A Manual of Psychological Medicine*, 1858 ed. 167–40.
15. Grimes, *Institutional Care*, 30. According to Grimes, the publication of these findings was blocked by the American Psychiatric Association; he published the study at his own expense. See especially v–xv, and also Albert Deutsch, *The Shame of the States* (New York, 1948), 102. See also Leonard Edelstein, *We Are Accountable: A View of Mental Institutions* (Wallingford, Pennsylvania, 1945), 7–11; "Casualties, Fatal Injuries, and Suicides in Hospitals for the Insane," *American Journal of Insanity*, 67 (1911), 607–09; and C. A. Bonner and Lois E. Taylor, "A Study of Accidents in a Mental Hospital," *American Journal of Psychiatry*, 18 (1939), 283–95.
16. George K. Butterfield, "What Happened to Discharged Patients?" *American Journal of Psychiatry*, 1 (1921), 177–82. See also Maurice C. Ashley, "Outcome of 1,000 Cases Paroled from the Middletown State Homeopathic Hospital," *State Hospital Quarterly*, 8 (1922–23), 64–70; William C. Garvin, "How the Number of Parole Patients Were Increased at the King's Park State Hospital,"

*State Hospital Quarterly*, 6 (1920–21), 67–76; and George W. Mills, "The Activities of a Parole Clinic," *State Hospital Quarterly*, 6 (1921–22), 215–35.

17. Charles F. Reed and David B. Rotman, "Study of Institutional Escapes," *American Journal of Psychiatry*, 2 (1922), 75, 86.

18. Jacob Kasanin and Esther C. Cook, "A Study of One Hundred Cases Discharged 'Against Advice' from the Boston Psychopathic Hospital in 1925," *Mental Hygiene*, 15 (1931), 155–71.

19. Horatio M. Pollock, *Mental Diseases and Social Welfare* (New York, 1933), 224–30. See also Pollock, "Is the Paroled Patient a Menace to the Community," *Psychiatric Quarterly*, 12 (1938), 236–44; Louis H. Cohen and Henry Freeman, "How Dangerous to the Community Are State Hospital Patients?" *Connecticut State Medical Journal*, 9 (1945), 697–99.

20. White, *Insanity and the Criminal Law* (New York, 1923), 27. For other accounts of the history of medical criminology, see especially Bromberg, *Psychiatry between the Wars*, 102–22; and Seymour Halleck, "American Psychiatry and the Criminal: A Historical Review," *American Journal of Psychiatry*, 121 (1965) 185–208. See also Thomas Szasz's appraisal in *Law, Liberty, and Psychiatry*, 171–241.

21. "New York's Crime Clinic," *American Journal of Psychiatry*, 11 (1932), 821. See also Frederic H. Leavitt, "Psychiatry and the Criminal," *American Journal of Psychiatry*, 89 (1932), 541–54; William Nelson, "Psychiatry and Its Relationship to the Administration of the Criminal Law," *American Journal of Psychiatry*, 89 (1933), 703–23; Lowell S. Selling, "A Psychiatric Technique for the Examination of Criminals," 93 (1937), 1097–1108; Matthew Molitch, "Chronic Post-Encephalitis in Juvenile Delinquents," *American Journal of Psychiatry*, 91 (1935), 842–61; and Menas S. Gregory, "Psychiatry and the Problems of Delinquency," *American Journal of Psychiatry*, 14 (1935), 773–81.

22. See Karpman's principal work, *Case Studies in the Psychopathology of Crime* (Washington, D.C., 1933). See also Karpman, "Psychosis in Criminals: Clinical Studies in the Psychopathology of Crime," *Journal of Nervous and Mental Disease*, 64 (1926), 331–51; Karpman, "Problem of Psychopathies," *Psychiatric Quarterly*, 3 (1929), 495–525; and Karpman, "Impulsive Neuroses and Crime; A Critical Review," *Journal of the American Institute of Criminal Law and Criminology*, 19 (1929), 575–91.

23. Bromberg, *Psychiatry between the Wars*, 105. See also Charles P. Bancroft, "Ought Limited Responsibility Be Recognized by the Courts?" *American Journal of Insanity*, 74 (1917), 139–48; Carlos F. MacDonald, "Should the Plea of Insanity as an Indictment for Crime Be Abolished?" *American Journal of Insanity*, 76 (1920), 295–302; F. J. Farnell, "The State, the Psychotic, and the Criminal," *Journal of Nervous and Mental Disease*, 72 (1930), 34–35; Bernard Glueck et al., "Psychiatry and Criminal Law," *Journal of Nervous and Mental Disease*, 81 (1935), 192–212; and Rollin M. Perkins, "Partial Insanity," *Journal of Criminal Law and Criminology*, 25 (1934), 175–86.

24. Bowers, "The Criminal Insane and the Insane Criminal," *American Journal of Insanity*, 74 (1917), 79.

25. William J. Nolan, "Some Characteristics of the Criminal Insane," *State Hospital Quarterly*, 5 (1919–20), 378.

26. Ellen Pilcher, "Relation of Mental Disease to Crime," *Journal of the American*

*Institute of Criminal Law and Criminology,* 21 (1930), 236. Most of the 392 patients with *dementia praecox* were committed because of the crime of disorderly conduct.

27. A. W. Stearns, "The Kind of Men in State Prison," *Journal of Abnormal Psychology,* 15 (1921), 335–49. See also "The Dangerous Insane," *Journal of the American Institute of Criminology,* 12 (1921–22), 369–80; Max A. Bahr, "Mental Reaction in Insane Criminal Behavior," *Medico-Legal Journal,* 42 (1925), 164–68; Albert Warren Stearns, "Homicide in Massachusetts," *American Journal of Psychiatry,* 4 (1925), 725–49; F. C. Shaw, "Types of Criminal Insane," *Psychiatric Quarterly,* 4 (1930), 458–65; F. R. Yeomans, "Who Are the 'Criminal Insane'? Fifty Patients Committed to Boston State Hospital," *Mental Hygiene,* 14 (1930), 672–96; T. J. Orbison, "Murderers' Row: Neuropsychiatric Study of Pathologic Behavior of 25 Murderers Who Killed 33 Persons," *California and Western Medicine,* 39 (1933), 104–09; Pilcher, "Relation of Mental Disease to Crime," 212–46; Charles A. Rymer, "The Insanity Plea in Murder," *American Journal of Psychiatry,* 21 (1942), 690–97; and Aaron J. Rosanoff, "Thirty Condemned Men," *American Journal of Psychiatry,* 21 (1942), 484–95.

## Chapter 8: Somatic and Dynamic Dangerousness, 1910–1960

1. Menninger, *The Vital Balance,* 466.
2. *Ibid.,* 464–86. Menninger notes that by 1917 the term "psychosis" was generally equated with mental illness requiring commitment.
3. Rosanoff, *Manual of Psychiatry,* 6th ed. (New York, 1927), 125. See also Archibald Church and Frederick Peterson, *Nervous and Mental Diseases,* 9th ed. (Philadelphia, 1919), 741, 754, 813; Edward A. Strecker and Franklin G. Ebaugh, *Practical Clinical Psychiatry* (Philadelphia, 1925), 238.
4. Church and Peterson, *Nervous and Mental Diseases,* 1919 ed., 599. Peterson was an opponent of dynamic psychiatry. In this edition, he reiterated: "There is no insanity without disease of the cortex. The material disorder of the cortex is diffuse and partly organic, but mostly functional in character. We term it functional, for thus far our pathologicoanatomical and clinical studies have failed to reveal any definite material bases for the majority of psychoses." 737.
5. White, *Outlines of Psychiatry,* 7th ed. (Washington, D.C., 1919), 174.
6. Church and Peterson, *Nervous and Mental Diseases,* 1919 ed., 599.
7. Glueck, *Mental Disorder and the Criminal Law* (Boston, 1925), 23.
8. William Alanson White and Smith Ely Jelliffe, eds., *Modern Treatment of Mental and Nervous Diseases* (Philadelphia, 1913), 217.
9. *Ibid.,* 592.
10. Noyes, *Modern Clinical Psychiatry* (Philadelphia, 1934), 229.
11. Strecker and Ebaugh, *Practical Clinical Psychiatry,* 4th ed. (Philadelphia, 1935), 373.
12. Bromberg, *Crime and the Mind: An Outline of Psychiatric Criminology,* (Philadelphia, 1948), 62.
13. John Holland Cassity, *The Quality of Murder: A Psychiatric and Legal Evaluation* (New York, 1958), 66, 73.
14. White and Jelliffe, *Diseases of the Nervous System,* 5th ed. (Philadelphia, 1929),

1039–42. See also Aaron J. Rosanoff, *Manual of Psychiatry*, 7th ed. (New York, 1938), 549–50; Samuel Henry Kraines, *The Therapy of Neuroses and Psychoses: A Socio-Psycho-Biologic Analysis and Resynthesis* (Philadelphia, 1941), 220–21; Oskar Diethelm, *Treatment in Psychiatry*, 2nd ed. (Springfield, Illinois, 1950), 235; Joseph L. Fetterman, *Practical Lessons in Psychiatry* (Springfield, Illinois, 1949), 142–45; Arthur P. Noyes and Lawrence C. Kolb, *Modern Clinical Psychiatry*, 5th ed. (Philadelphia, 1958), 400; A. W. Hackfield, "Crimes of Unintelligible Motivation as Representing an Insidiously Developing Schizophrenia," *American Journal of Psychiatry* 14 (1934), 642–43; and Lowell S. Selling, "The Psychopathology of the Hit and Run Driver," *American Journal of Psychiatry*, 21 (1941), 97.

15. Arieti, "Schizophrenia: Symptomatology and Mechanisms," in Arieti, ed., *American Handbook of Psychiatry* (New York, 1959), 461; Strecker and Ebaugh, *Practical Clinical Psychiatry*, 1935 ed., 399.

16. White and Jelliffe, *Modern Treatment of Mental and Nervous Diseases*, 1913 ed., 631–32.

17. Church and Peterson, *Nervous and Mental Diseases*, 1919 ed., 840. See also Strecker and Ebaugh, *Practical Clinical Psychiatry*, 1935 ed., 427; White, *Outlines of Psychiatry*, 1919 ed., 92–93; and Noyes, *Modern Clinical Psychiatry*, 175–78.

18. Church and Peterson, *Nervous and Mental Diseases*, 1919 ed., 840. See also Flemming, "The Murder of Dr. George F. Lloyd," 295.

19. White and Jelliffe, *Modern Treatment of Mental and Nervous Diseases*, 1913 ed., 621.

20. White, *Outlines of Psychiatry*, 1919 ed., 93.

21. Noyes, *Modern Clinical Psychiatry*, 187.

22. White and Jelliffe, *Modern Treatment*, 1929 ed., 233. See also Diethelm, *Treatment in Psychiatry*, 270–71; Noyes and Kolb, *Modern Clinical Psychiatry*, 1958 ed., 446; Strecker and Ebaugh, *Practical Clinical Psychiatry*, 1940 ed., 456; Thomas Butterworth and Joseph McIver, "Paranoia with Report of a Case," *American Journal of Psychiatry*, 10 (1930), 268; and Norman Cameron, "Paranoid Conditions and Paranoia," in Arieti, *American Handbook of Psychiatry*, 1959 ed., 520.

23. White and Jelliffe, *Modern Treatment*, 1913 ed., 232–33. See also Karpman, "The Myth of the Psychopathic Personality," *American Journal of Psychiatry*, 104 (1948), 523–24.

24. Karpman, "The Psychopathic Individual: A Symposium," *Mental Hygiene*, 8 (1924), 199. See also Henry Werlinder, *Psychopathy: A History of the Concept* (Stockholm, 1978), 131–70; Pierre Pichot, "Psychopathic Behavior: A Historical Overview," in R. D. Hare and D. Schalling, *Psychopathic Behavior: Approaches to Research* (New York, 1978), 55–70; White, *Outlines of Psychiatry*, 1919 ed., 270; Strecker and Ebaugh, *Practical Clinical Psychiatry*, 1935 ed., 328–41, 467–82; and Noyes, *Modern Clinical Psychiatry*, 434–50.

25. Menninger, *The Vital Balance*, 460–61. See also Rosanoff, *Manual of Psychiatry*, 1927 ed., 187; James V. May, *Mental Diseases: A Public Health Problem* (Boston, 1922), 511–23; J. H. Huddleston, "The Part of Conduct Disorders in the Concept of Constitutional Psychopathic Inferiority," *Journal of Nervous and Mental Disease*, 64 (1926), 151–56; G. E. Partridge, "A Study of 50 Cases of Psychopathic Personality," *American Journal of Psychiatry*, 7 (1928), 953–73;

and Partridge, "Current Conceptions of Psychopathic Personality," *American Journal of Psychiatry*, 10 (1930), 53–79.

26. Noyes, *Modern Clinical Psychiatry*, 1934 ed., 441.

27. Rosanoff, *Manual of Psychiatry*, 1927 ed., 189–90.

28. Kraines, *The Therapy of Neuroses and Psychoses*, 1948 ed., 511–12.

29. Yawger, "Is There a 'Moral Center' in the Brain?" *American Journal of the Medical Sciences*, 189 (1935), 265.

30. Noyes and Kolb, *Modern Clinical Psychiatry*, 1958 ed., 549. See, however, R. H. Bryant, "The Constitutional Psychopathic Inferior a Menace to Society and a Suggestion for the Disposition of Such Individuals," *American Journal of Psychiatry*, 6 (1927), 671–89.

31. Alfred Gordon, "Medico-Legal Aspects of Morbid Impulses," *New York Medical Journal and Medical Record*, 65 (1922), 617.

32. Dercum, *A Clinical Manual of Mental Diseases*, 2nd ed. (Philadelphia, 1917), 195. See also Karpman, "Impulsive Neuroses and Crime: A Critical Review," 575–91; and Jacob Goldwyn, "Impulses to Incendiarism and Theft," *American Journal of Psychiatry*, 87 (1930), 1093–99.

33. White and Jelliffe, *Modern Treatment of Mental and Nervous Diseases*, 1913 ed., 408.

34. White, *Outlines of Psychiatry*, 1919 ed., 74–77.

35. Ibid., 264–68. See also Strecker and Ebaugh, *Practical Clinical Psychiatry*, 1935 ed., 549–56; and Noyes, *Modern Clinical Psychiatry*, 104–05.

36. Menninger, *The Vital Balance*, 236–40. Menninger classified all forms of dangerous insanity as "A Third Order of Dyscontrol." For his dynamic analysis of dangerousness, see pp. 213–49. See also Noyes, *Modern Clinical Psychiatry*, 104–05, 414–23; Noyes and Kolb, *Modern Clinical Psychiatry*, 391, 413, 420, 526; Paul H. Hoch and Philip Polalin, "Pseudoneurotic Forms of Schizophrenia," *Psychiatric Quarterly*, 23 (1949), 248–50; Richard W. Nice, ed., *Crime and Insanity* (New York, 1958), 29–48; Cassity, *The Quality of Murder*, 95–111; John Frosch and S. B. Wortis, "A Contribution to the Nosology of the Impulse Disorders," *American Journal of Psychiatry*, (1954), 132–38; and Joseph Satten et al., "Murder Without Apparent Motive," *American Journal of Psychiatry*, 117 (1960), 48–53.

37. White and Jelliffe, *Modern Treatment of Mental and Nervous Diseases*, 1913 ed., 216.

38. Temkin, *The Falling Sickness*, 351–59. See also Church and Peterson, *Nervous and Mental Diseases*, 1919 ed., 658–59; Noyes, *Modern Clinical Psychiatry*, 235; C. Kirk, "Analysis of More than 200 Cases of Epilepsy Treated with Luminal," *American Journal of Insanity*, 77 (1921), 559–63; Mary L. Austin, *The Use of Luminal in Epilepsy* (Columbus, Ohio, 1922); Ewen D. Cameron, "The Dehydration Method in Epilepsy," *American Journal of Psychiatry*, 11 (1931), 123–30; Douglas A. Thom, "Epilepsy and Its Rational Extrainstitutional Treatment," *American Journal of Psychiatry*, 10 (1931), 623–35; Foster Kennedy, "Clinical Convulsions," *American Journal of Psychiatry*, 11 (1932), 601–09; Calvert Stein, "Studies in Endocrine Therapy in Epilepsy," *American Journal of Psychiatry*, 13 (1934), 739–60, 16 (1937), 1181–83; William C. Lennox, "The Campaign against Epilepsy," *American Journal of Psychiatry*, 17 (1937), 251–62; and Moe Moldstein, "Results of 15 Years Experience with the Ketogenic

Diet in the Treatment of Epilepsy in Children," *American Journal of Psychiatry*, 17 (1938), 1205–14.

39. Eugen Bleuler, *Textbook of Psychiatry*, trans. A. A. Brill (New York, 1924), 448–49. See also Noyes, *Modern Clinical Psychiatry*, 236; Strecker and Ebaugh, *Practical Clinical Psychiatry*, 1935 ed., 166; White, *Outlines of Psychiatry*, 1919 ed., 242–43; and Rosanoff, *Manual of Psychiatry*, 1927 ed., 90.

40. Bridge, "Mental State of the Epileptic Patient," *Archives of Neurology and Psychiatry*, 32 (1934), 736. See also Diethelm, "Epileptic Convulsions and the Personality Setting," *Archives of Neurology and Psychiatry*, 31 (1934), 755; and R. A. Clark and J. M. Lesko, "Psychosis Associated with Epilepsy," *American Journal of Psychiatry*, 19 (1939), 595–607.

41. Paine, "Psychotic Symptoms of Epilepsy," *American Journal of Psychiatry*, 2 (1923), 716. See also H. S. Gregory, "The Problem of the Epileptic Insane," *State Hospital Quarterly*, 6 (1920–21), 355–56.

42. Herbert H. Jasper and Ira C. Nichols, "Electrical Signs of Cortical Function in Epilepsy and Allied Disorders," *American Journal of Psychiatry*, 17 (1938), 835–51. See also, for example, two early studies: Norman Q. Brill, "Electroencephalographic Studies in Delinquent Behavior Problem Children," *American Journal of Psychiatry*, 21 (1942), 494–98; and Warren T. Brown and Charles I. Solomon, "Delinquency and the Electroencephalograph," *American Journal of Psychiatry*, 21 (1942), 499–503.

43. H. H. Merritt and T. J. Putnam, "Sodium Diphenthydantoinate in the Treatment of Convulsive Disorders," *Journal of the American Medical Association*, 111 (1938), 1068–73; "Council on Acceptance Report," *Journal of the American Medical Association*, 113 (1939), 1734; Willard W. Dickerson, "The Present Status of Dilantin Therapy," *American Journal of Psychiatry*, 21 (1942), 515–23.

44. John M. MacDonald, *Psychiatry and the Criminal*, 3rd ed. (Springfield, Illinois, 1976), 222–24. See also T. A. Betts, H. Mersky, and D. A. Pond, "Psychiatry," in John Laidlow and Alan Richens, eds., *A Textbook of Epilepsy* (Edinburgh, 1976), 175–76; Hans Strauss, "Epileptic Disorders," in Arieti, *American Handbook of Psychiatry*, 1959 ed., 1114, 1121–22; and Ira Sherwin, "Neurobiological Basis of Psychopathology Associated with Epilepsy," in Harry Sands, ed., *Epilepsy: A Handbook for the Mental Health Professional* (New York, 1982), 77–96.

45. Harrower-Erickson, "Psychological Studies of Patients with Epileptic Seizures," in Wilder Penfield and Theodore C. Erickson, *Epilepsy and Cerebral Localization* (Springfield, Illinois, 1941), 546–74.

## Chapter 9: Prediction, Confidentiality, and the Duty to Warn

1. Frank T. Lindman and Donald M. McIntyre, Jr., eds., *The Mentally Disabled and the Law* (Chicago, 1961). See also Ronald S. Rock, Marcus A. Jacobson, and Richard M. Janopaul, eds., *Hospitalization and Discharge of the Mentally Ill* (Chicago, 1968), 77–120.

2. Shah, "Dangerousness and Mental Illness: Some Conceptual, Prediction, and

Policy Dilemmas," in Calvin J. Frederick, *Dangerous Behavior: A Problem in Law and Mental Health* (Rockville, Maryland, 1978), 155.

3. Brooks, "Notes on Defining 'Dangerousness' of the Mentally Ill," in Frederick, *Dangerous Behavior*, 41. For a list of the more important legal decisions, see Calvin J. Frederick, "An Overview of Dangerousness: Its Complexities and Consequences," in Frederick, *Dangerous Behavior*, 10.

4. "Developments in the Law: Civil Commitment of the Mentally Ill," *Harvard Law Review*, 87 (1974), 1190, 1207–12. For a summary of these statutes, see Bruce Ennis and Loren Siegel, *The Rights of Mental Patients: The Basic ACLU Guide to a Mental Patient's Rights* (New York, 1973), 93–282.

5. Jonas R. Rappeport, George Lassen, and Nancy B. Hay, "A Review of the Literature on the Dangerousness of the Mentally Ill," in Rappeport, ed., *The Clinical Evaluation of Dangerousness in the Mentally Ill* (Washington, D.C., 1967), 72–80. See also Shah, "Dangerousness and Mental Illness: Some Conceptual, Prediction, and Policy Dilemmas," 165–58; and Ennis and Siegel, *The Basic ACLU Guide to a Mental Patient's Rights*, 287–90.

6. Rappeport and Lassen, "Dangerousness: Arrest Rate Comparison of Discharged Patients and the General Population," *American Journal of Psychiatry*, 121 (1965), 776–83; Rappeport and Lassen, "The Dangerousness of Female Patients: A Comparison of the Arrest Rate of Discharged Psychiatric Patients and the General Population," *American Journal of Psychiatry*, 123 (1966), 413–19.

7. See for example, A. Zitrin et al., "Crime and Violence among Mental Patients," *American Journal of Psychiatry*, 133 (1976), 142–49.

8. Shah, "Dangerousness and Mental Illness: Some Conceptual, Prediction, and Policy Dilemmas," 161. See also John M. MacDonald, *Homicidal Threats* (Springfield, Illinois, 1968), 21–35.

9. Frederic Grunberg, Burton I. Klinger, and Barbara Brumet, "Homicide and Deinstitutionalization of the Mentally Ill," *American Journal of Psychiatry*, 134 (1977), 687. See also Heinz E. Lehmann, "Schizophrenia: Clinical Features," in Freedman, Kaplan, and Sadock, *Comprehensive Textbook of Psychiatry/III*, 2, 1178.

10. Henry J. Steadman and Joseph J. Cocozza, *Careers of the Criminally Insane* (Lexington, Massachusetts, 1974). See also T. P. Thornberry and J. E. Jacoby, *The Criminally Insane* (Chicago, 1979). For a summary of Steadman and Cocozza's prediction research, see Steadman, "Special Problems in the Prediction of Violence among the Mentally Ill," in J. Ray Hays, Thomm Kevin Roberts, and Kenneth S. Solway, eds., *Violence and the Violent Individual* (New York, 1981), 243–56.

11. Stephen J. Pfohl, *Predicting Dangerousness* (Lexington, Massachusetts, 1978), 106.

12. Paul E. Meehl, *Clinical versus Statistical Prediction: A Theoretical Analysis and Review of the Literature* (Minneapolis, 1954). See also Martin L. Forst, "The Psychiatric Evaluation of Dangerousness in Two Trial Court Jurisdictions," *Bulletin of the American Academy of Psychiatry and Law*, 6 (1977), 102–08.

13. *Task Force Report* 8, 30.

14. See, for example, Grunberg, Klinger, and Grumet, "Homicide and Deinstitutionalization of the Mentally Ill," 685–87. See also John Monahan, "Pre-

diction Research and the Emergency Commitment of Dangerous Mentally Ill Persons: A Reconsideration," *American Journal of Psychiatry*, 135 (1978), 198.

15. *Task Force Report* 8, 2. Compare with Ray, *A Treatise on the Medical Jurisprudence of Insanity*, 1838 ed., 232–33.
16. *Task Force Report* 8, 8.
17. *Ibid.*, The Task Force rejected the XYZ variant as a biological predictor.
18. *Ibid.*
19. Strecker and Ebaugh, *Practical Clinical Psychiatry*, 5th ed. (Philadelphia, 1940), 456. See also Lawrence C. Kolb, *Noyes' Modern Clinical Psychiatry*, 8th ed., (Philadelphia, 1973), 392.
20. Rado, "Obsessive Behavior: A So-Called Obsessive-Compulsive Neurosis," in Arieti, *American Handbook of Psychiatry*, 1974 ed., 194–208.
21. Alfred M. Freedman, Harold I. Kaplan, and Benjamin J. Sadock, *Modern Synopsis of Comprehensive Textbook of Psychiatry/II*, 2nd ed. (Baltimore, 1976), 397,490.
22. Max Day and Elvin V. Semrad, "Paranoia and Paranoid States," in Armand M. Nicholi, Jr., ed., *The Harvard Guide to Modern Psychiatry*, 2nd ed. (Cambridge, Massachusetts, 1978), 243–52. See also J. Ingram Walker and H. Keith H. Brodie, "Paranoid Disorders," in Freeman, Kaplan, and Sadock, *Comprehensive Textbook of Psychiatry/III*, 1980 ed., 1921.
23. Kolb, *Modern Clinical Psychiatry*, 1973, 429. See also Freedman, Kaplan, and Sadock, *Modern Synopsis*, 633.
24. Freedman, Kaplan, and Sadock, *Modern Synopsis*, 451.
25. Max Day and Elvin V. Semrad, "Schizophrenic Reactions," in Nicholi, *The Harvard Guide to Modern Psychiatry*, 213. See also Lehmann, "Schizophrenia: Clinical Features," 1177.
26. Kolb, *Noyes' Modern Clinical Psychiatry*, 1973 ed., 498.
27. MacDonald, *Psychiatry and the Criminal*, 1975 ed., 281.
28. The literature on this subject is extensive. The most comprehensive sources on all facets of human violence are: William S. Fields and William H. Sweet, eds., *Neural Basis of Violence and Aggression* (St. Louis, 1975). See pages 277–79 for a description of the "epileptic personality."
29. Ervin and Mark, *Violence and the Brain*. See also Vernon H. Mark, William Sweet, and Frank Ervin, "Deep Temporal Lobe Stimulation and Destructive Lesions in Episodically Violent Temporal Lobe Epileptics," in Fields and Sweet, *Neural Basis of Violence and Aggression*, 379–91. This kind of work on the human brain has not been accepted without controversy within the medical profession. See especially Peter Roger Breggin, "Psychosurgery for the Control of Violence: A Critical Review." Breggin, Executive Director for the Study of Psychiatry, Washington, D.C., was chosen as spokesperson for a group of physicians who protested the use of psychosurgery on the mentally ill and prisoners. In this paper, Breggin targeted Ervin and Mark's work and questioned both the adequacy of their experimental methods and the ethics involved in the experiments on human subjects.
30. Stone, "Psychiatry and the Law," in Nicholi, *The Harvard Guide to Modern Psychiatry*, 1978 ed., 654.
31. *Task Force Report* 8, 33.

32. *Ibid.*, 32.
33. See, for example, Philip Solomon and Vernon D. Patch, *Handbook of Psychiatry*, 3rd ed. (Los Altos, California, 1974), 408–19. See also W. L. Linford Rees, *A Short Textbook of Psychiatry* (London, 1976), 281; John R. Lion and Denis Madden, "Management of the Violent Patient," in George U. Balis et al., *Psychiatric Problems in Medical Practice: The Psychiatric Foundations of Medicine* (Boston, 1978), 265–73; Andrew A. Slaby, Julian Lieb, and Laurence R. Tancredi, *Handbook of Psychiatric Emergencies*, 2nd ed. (New York, 1981), 168–72; and Steven L. Dudovsky and Michael P. Weissberg, *Clinical Psychiatry in Primary Care* (Baltimore, 1982), 262–63.
34. Tarasoff v. Regents of the University of California et al., 131 Cal, Rptr 14, 551, p2d, 334 (Cal 1976).
35. Paul S. Appelbaum, "*Tarasoff* and the Clinician: Problems in Fulfilling the Duty to Protect," *American Journal of Psychiatry*, 142 (1985), 425–29.

# Bibliography

## Primary Sources

### Annual Reports (listed by state; titles vary)

Connecticut Retreat for the Insane. Hartford, Connecticut. 1826–74.
General Hospital for the Insane. Middletown, Connecticut. 1852–1900.
Government Hospital for the Insane. Washington, D.C. 1855–91.
Maine Insane Hospital. Augusta, Maine. 1840–1900.
Mount Hope Hospital. Baltimore, Maryland. 1843–82.
Boston Lunatic Asylum. South Boston, Massachusetts. 1839–54.
Massachusetts General Hospital, McLean Asylum. Boston, Massachusetts. 1823–1901.
State Lunatic Hospital. Worcester, Massachusetts. 1833–1900.
New Hampshire Asylum for the Insane. Concord, New Hampshire. 1842–1900.
State of New York, Commission in Lunacy. 1889–1910.
New York State Lunatic Asylum. Utica, New York. 1843–1906.
State of New York, State Board of Charities. 1867–96.
Asylum for the Insane. Athens, Ohio. 1873–1900.
Northern Ohio Lunatic Asylum. Cleveland, Ohio. 1854–1900.
Ohio Hospital for Epileptics. Gallipolis, Ohio. 1890–1909.
Ohio Lunatic Asylum. Columbus, Ohio. 1841–1902.
The Asylum for the Relief of Persons Deprived of the Use of Their Reason. Frankfort, Pennsylvania. 1851–88.
State Lunatic Asylum. Harrisburg, Pennsylvania. 1851–1900.
Eastern Lunatic Asylum. Williamsburg, Virginia. 1868–83.
Western Lunatic Asylum. Staunton, Virginia. 1851–70.
West Virginia Hospital for the Insane. Weston, West Virginia. 1864–78.

## Psychiatric Serials

*Alienist and Neurologist.* 1880–1920.
*American Journal of Insanity.* 1844–1921.
*American Journal of Neurology and Psychiatry.* 1882–85.
*American Journal of Psychiatry.* 1921–85.
*Archives of Neurology and Psychiatry.* 1919–83.
*Journal of Mental Science.* 1854–1910.
*Journal of Nervous and Mental Disease.* 1874–1983
*Mental Hygiene.* 1917–83.
*Quarterly Journal of Psychological Medicine and Medical Jurisprudence.* 1867–69.
*State Hospital Bulletin.* 1896–97.
*State Hospital Quarterly.* 1915–26.

## Articles

Allbutt, C., "Homicidal Insanity," *Lancet,* 197 (1919), 34.

Allen, J. A., "Case of Homicidal Monomania," *Boston Medical and Surgical Journal,* 39 (1850), 441–46.

"Automatic Homicide," *British Medical Journal,* January 2, 1886, 26.

Bahr, Max A., "Mental Reaction in Insane Criminal Behavior," *Medico-Legal Journal,* 42 (1925), 164–68.

Baudry, J. K., "Epilepsy in Its Medico-Legal Relations to the Case of Max Klingler," *St. Louis Medical and Surgical Journal,* (1870), 507.

Blachly, P. H., and D. Gowing, "Multiple Monitored Electroconvulsive Treatment," *Comprehensive Psychiatry,* 7 (1966), 100–10.

Bowers, Paul E., "The Dangerous Insane," *Journal of the American Institute of Criminology,* 12 (1921–22), 369–80.

Brigham, Amariah, "Case of Homicidal Insanity," *Phrenological Journal of Edinburgh,* 17 (1844), 32.

Brill, A. A., "Psychological Mechanisms in Paranoia," *New York Medical Journal,* 94 (1911), 957–74.

Butts, A.C., "Killing of Children by Insane Parents," *Medico-Legal Journal,* 4 (1886–87), 37–48.

Carr, W. W., "The Webber Murder Case in Philadelphia," *Medico-Legal Journal,* 4 (1886–89), 243–62.

Channing, Walter, "The Use of Mechanical Restraint," *Boston Medical and Surgical Journal,* 103 (1880), 173–77.

Cohen, Louis H., and H. Freeman, "How Dangerous to the Community Are State Hospital Patients?" *Connecticut State Medical Journal,* 9 (1945), 697–99.

Conklin, W. J., "The Relations of Epilepsy to Insanity and Jurisprudence," address before the Ohio State Medical Society, April 6, 1871.

"Council on Acceptance Report," *Journal of the American Medical Association,* 113 (1939), 1734.

"Developments in the Law: Civil Commitment of the Mentally Ill," *Harvard Law Review* 87 (1974), 1190, 1207–12, 1222–23.

Elstun, W. J., "Hydrate of Chloral and Some of Its Effects in Insanity," *Indiana Journal of Medicine,* 1 (1871), 257–64.

Forst, Martin L., "The Psychiatric Evaluation of Dangerousness in Two Trial Court Jurisdictions," *Bulletin of the American Academy of Psychiatry and Law*, 6 (1977), 98–110.

Furlong, F. W., "The Mythology of Electroconvulsive Therapy," *Comprehensive Psychiatry*, 13 (1972), 235–40.

Gordon, Alfred, "Medicolegal Aspect of Morbid Impulses," *New York Medical Journal and Medical Record*, 65 (1922), 616–21.

Hamilton, Alan McLane, "The Development of the Legal Relations concerning the Insane, with Suggestions for Reform," *Medical Record*, 74 (1908), 781–88.

Hoch, Paul H., and Philip Polalin, "Pseudoneurotic Forms of Schizophrenia," *Psychiatric Quarterly*, 23 (1949), 248–56.

Hurwitz, Thomas D., "Electroconvulsive Therapy: A Review," *Comprehensive Psychiatry*, 15 (1974), 303–14.

"Insanity and Crime," *British Medical Journal*, 14 (1858), 404.

Karpman, Benjamin, "Impulsive Neuroses and Crime: Critical Review," *Journal of the American Institute of Criminal Law and Criminology*, 19 (1929), 575–91.

———. "Problem of Psychopathies," *Psychiatric Quarterly*, 3 (1929), 495–525.

Laird, S. Louise, "Nursing of the Insane," *American Journal of Nursing*, 2 (1902), 170–80.

Lence, W. C., "The Management and Treatment of the Insane," *Medical Review*, 34 (1896), 5–7.

Mann, Edward C., "The Legal Relations of Imbecility and of Suicidal and Homicidal Mania," *Brooklyn Medical Journal*, 4 (1890), 132–39.

Merritt, H. H., and T. J. Putnam, "Sodium Diphenyl Hydantoinate in the Treatment of Convulsive Disorders," *Journal of the American Medical Association*, 11 (1938), 1068–73.

Mesnikoff, Alvin M., and Carl G. Lauterbach, "The Association of Violent Dangerous Behavior with Psychiatric Disorders: A Review of the Research Literature," *Journal of Psychiatry and Law*, 3 (1975), 415–46.

Orbison, T. J., "Murderers' Row: Neuropsychiatric Study of Pathologic Behavior of 25 Murderers Who Killed 33 Persons," *California and Western Medicine*, 39 (1933), 104–09.

Perkins, Rollin M., "Partial Insanity," *Journal of Criminal Law and Criminology*, 25 (1934), 175–86.

Pilcher, Ellen, "Relation of Mental Disease to Crime," *Journal of the American Institute of Criminal Law and Criminology*, 21 (1930), 212–46.

Prince, Morton, "A Case of 'Imperative Idea' or 'Homicidal Impulse' in a Neurasthenic without Hereditary Taint," *Boston Medical and Surgical Journal*, 137 (1897), 57–58.

Shaw, F. C., "Types of Criminal Insane," *Psychiatric Quarterly*, 4 (1930), 458–65.

Spratling, W. P., "The Treatment of the Acutely Insane in General Hospitals," *Medical Record*, 37 (1890), 729.

Stearns, A. W., and J. V. Chapman, "The Kind of Men in State Prison," *Journal of Abnormal Psychology*, 15 (1921), 335–49.

Thayer, Addison S., "Five Maine Murders," *Boston Medical and Surgical Journal*, 146 (1902), 215–19.

Wilbur, H. B., "Chemical Restraint," *Archives of Medicine*, 6 (1881), 271–92.

Yawger, N. S., "Is there a 'Moral Center' in the Brain?" *American Journal of Medical Sciences*, 189 (1935), 265–70.

Yellowlees, David, "Homicidal Mania: A Biography with Physiological and Medico-Legal Comments," *Edinburgh Medical Journal*, 8 (1862–63), 105–24.

Zilboorg, Gregory, "Sidelights on Parent-Child Antagonism," *American Journal of Orthopsychiatry*, 2 (1932), 35–43.


*Books*


*Account of the Rise and Progress of the Asylum, Proposed to Be Established, near Philadelphia, for the Relief of Persons Deprived of the Use of their Reason, with an Abridged Account of the Retreat, a Similar Institution near York, England.* Philadelphia, 1814.

American Psychiatric Association. *Diagnostic and Statistical Manual of Mental Disorders.* 3rd ed. Washington, D.C., 1980.

———. *Task Force Report 8: Clinical Aspects of the Violent Individual.* Washington, D.C., 1974.

Arieti, Silvano, ed. *American Handbook of Psychiatry.* New York, 1959.

———. *American Handbook of Psychiatry.* 2nd ed. New York, 1974.

Austin, Mary L. *The Use of Luminal in Epilepsy.* Columbus, Ohio, 1922.

Balis, George U., et al. *Psychiatric Problems in Medical Practice: The Psychiatric Foundations of Medicine.* Boston, 1978.

Bayle, A. L. J. *Recherches sur les malades mentales.* Paris, 1822.

Beard, George M. *A Practical Treatise on Nervous Exhaustion (Neurasthenia): Its Symptoms, Nature, Sequences, Treatment.* New York, 1880.

Beck, Theodric Romeyn. *Elements of Medical Jurisprudence.* 3rd ed. London, 1829.

———. *Inaugural Dissertation on Insanity.* New York, 1811.

Beck, Theodric Romeyn, and John B. Beck. *Elements of Medical Jurisprudence.* 2 vols. 11th ed. Philadelphia, 1860.

Bevan-Lewis, W. *A Text-Book of Mental Diseases.* 2nd ed. London 1899.

Blandford, G. Fielding. *Insanity and Its Treatment.* 3rd ed. New York, 1886.

Bleuler, Eugen. *Textbook of Psychiatry.* Trans. A. A. Brill. New York, 1924.

Brigham, Amariah. *An Inquiry Concerning the Diseases and Functions of Brain, the Spinal Cord, and the Nerves.* New York, 1840.

Bromberg, Walter. *Crime and the Mind: An Outline of Psychiatric Criminology.* Philadelphia, 1948.

Bucknill, John Charles. *The Care of the Insane and Their Legal Control.* 2nd ed. London, 1880.

———. *Unsoundness of Mind in Relation to Criminal Acts*, 2nd ed. London, 1857.

Bucknill, John Charles, and Daniel Hack Tuke. *A Manual of Psychological Medicine.* London, 1858.

———. *A Manual of Psychological Medicine.* 2nd ed. London, 1862.

———. *A Manual of Psychological Medicine.* 3rd ed. London, 1874.

———. *A Manual of Psychological Medicine.* 4th ed. London, 1879.

———. *A Manual of Psychological Medicine.* 5th ed. London, 1880.

Burrows, George Mann. *Commentaries on the Causes, Forms, Symptoms, and Treatment, Moral and Medical, of Insanity.* London, 1828.

Cassity, John Holland. *The Quality of Murder: A Psychiatric and Legal Evaluation.* New York, 1958.

Church, Archibald, and Frederick Peterson. *Nervous and Mental Diseases.* 3rd ed. Philadelphia, 1901.

———. *Nervous and Mental Diseases.* 9th ed. Philadelphia, 1919.

Clark, L. Pierce. *Epilepsy and the Convulsive State.* Baltimore, 1931.

Clouston, Thomas Smith. *Clinical Lectures on Mental Disease.* London, 1883: Philadelphia, 1884.

———. *Clinical Lectures on Mental Disease.* 6th ed. London, 1904.

Cobb, Stanley. *Foundations of Neuropsychiatry.* 2nd. ed. Baltimore, 1941.

Combe, Andrew. *Observations on Mental Derangement: Being an Application of the Principles of Phrenology to the Elucidation of the Causes, Symptoms, Nature, and Treatment of Insanity.* Boston, 1834.

Commission on Lunacy [Levi Lincoln, Edward Jarvis, and Increase Sumner]. *Report on Insanity and Idiocy in Massachusetts.* Boston, 1855.

Conklin, W. J. *The Relations of Epilepsy to Insanity and Jurisprudence* (address before the Ohio State Medical Society). April 6, 1871.

Conolly, John. *An Inquiry concerning the Indications of Insanity with Suggestions for the Better Protection and Care of the Insane.* London, 1830.

———. *Treatment of the Insane without Mechanical Restraints.* London, 1856.

Dana, Charles, L. *A Textbook of Nervous Diseases and Psychiatry.* 6th ed. New York, 1904.

Defendorf [Diefendorf], A. Ross. *Clinical Psychiatry: A Text-Book for Students and Physicians, Abstracted and Adapted from the Sixth German Edition of Kraepelin's "Lehrbuch der Psychiatrie."* New York, 1902.

Dercum, Francis X. *A Clinical Manual of Mental Diseases.* 2nd ed. Philadelphia, 1917.

Diefendorf, A. Ross. *Clinical Psychiatry: A Text-Book for Students and Physicians, Abstracted and Adapted from the Sixth German Edition of Kraepelin's "Lehrbuch der Psychiatrie."* 2nd ed. New York, 1912.

Deutsch, Albert. *The Shame of the States.* New York, 1948.

Diethelm, Oskar. *Treatment in Psychiatry.* 2nd ed. Springfield, Illinois, 1950.

Dudovsky, Steven L., and Michael P. Weissberg. *Clinical Psychiatry in Primary Care.* Baltimore, 1982.

Earle, Pliny. *A Visit to Thirteen Asylums for the Insane in Europe with an Essay on Insanity.* Philadelphia, 1841.

Echeverria, Manuel Gonzalez. *On Epilepsy: Anatomo-Pathological and Clinical Notes.* New York, 1870.

Eddy, Thomas, *Hints for Introducing an Approved Mode of Treating the Insane in the Asylum.* New York, 1815.

Edelstein, Leonard. *We Are Accountable: A View of Mental Institutions.* Wallingford, Pennsylvania, 1945.

Ennis, Bruce, and Loren Siegel. *The Rights of Mental Patients: The Basic ACLU Guide to a Mental Patient's Rights.* New York, 1973.

Esquirol, J. E. D. *Des maladies mentales.* Paris, 1828.

———. *Observations on the Illusions of the Insane and upon the Medico-Legal Question of their Confinement.* Trans. William Liddell. London, 1833.

Fetterman, Joseph L. *Practical Lessons in Psychiatry.* Springfield, Illinois, 1949.

Fields, William S., and William H. Sweet, eds. *Neural Basis of Violence and Aggression*. St. Louis, 1975.
Frederick, Calvin J. *Dangerous Behavior: A Problem in Law and Mental Health*. Rockville, Maryland, 1978.
Franz, Shepherd Ivory. *Handbook of Mental Examination Methods*. New York, 1912.
Freedman, Alfred M. Harold I. Kaplan and Benjamin J. Sadock. *Comprehensive Textbook of Psychiatry/III*. 3 vols. 3rd ed. Baltimore, 1980.
———. *Modern Synopsis of Comprehensive Textbook of Psychiatry/II*. 2nd ed. Baltimore, 1976.
Georget, Étienne. *Discussion médico-légale sur la folie*. Paris, 1826.
Glueck, Sheldon. *Mental Disorder and the Criminal Law*. Boston, 1925.
Gowers, W. R. *Epilepsy and Other Chronic Convulsive Diseases: Their Causes, Symptoms, and Treatment*. New York, 1885.
———. *A Manual of Diseases of the Nervous System*. 2 vols. 2nd ed. Philadelphia, 1893.
Granger, William D. *How to Care for the Insane: A Manual for Attendants in Insane Asylums*. New York, 1886.
Greenblatt, Milton, and H. C. Solomin. *Frontal Lobes and Schizophrenia; Second Lobotomy Project of Boston Psychopathic Hospital*. New York, 1953.
Grimes, John Maurice. *Institutional Care of Mental Patients in the United States*. Chicago, 1934.
Gross, Samuel D., ed. *Lives of Eminent American Physicians and Surgeons of the Nineteenth Century*. Philadelphia, 1861.
Hamilton, Alan McLane. *Types of Insanity*. New York, 1886.
Hammond, William A. *Insanity in Its Relations to Crime*. New York, 1873.
———. *The Non-Asylum Treatment of the Insane*. New York, 1879.
———. *A Treatise on the Diseases of the Nervous System*. 6th ed. New York, 1876.
———. *A Treatise on Insanity in Its Medical Relations*. New York, 1883.
Hare, R. D., and D. Schalling. *Psychopathic Behavior: Approaches to Research*. New York, 1978.
Harrison, George L. *Legislation on Insanity*. Philadelphia, 1884.
Hays, J. Ray, Thomm Kevin Roberts, and Kenneth S. Solway, eds. *Violence and the Violent Individual*. New York, 1981.
Healy, William, and A. F. Bronner. *Delinquents and Criminals*. New York, 1926.
Henry, George W. *Essentials of Psychiatry*. 2nd ed. Baltimore, 1931.
Hirsch, Gordon L., ed. *The New Chemotherapy in Mental Illness*. New York, 1958.
Ingleby, David, ed. *Critical Psychiatry: The Politics of Mental Health*. New York, 1980.
Jackson, John Hughlings. *Clinical and Physiological Researches on the Nervous System*. London, 1875.
———. *Neurological Fragments*. London, 1925.
Jelliffe, Smith Ely. *A Summary of the Origins, Transformations, and Present-Day Trends of the Paranoia Concept*. New York, 1913.
Karpman, Benjamin. *Case Studies in the Psychopathology of Crime*. 15 vols. Washington, D.C., 1933–48.
Kellogg, Theodore H. *A Text-Book of Mental Diseases*. New York, 1897.
Kirchoff, Theodore. *Handbook of Insanity for Practitioners and Students*. New York, 1893.

Kirkbride, Thomas Story. *On the Construction, Organization, and General Arrangements of Hospitals for the Insane*. Philadelphia, 1854.
Kolb, Lawrence C. *Noyes' Modern Clinical Psychiatry*. 8th ed. Philadelphia, 1973.
———. *Noyes' Modern Clinical Psychiatry*. 9th ed. Philadelphia, 1981.
Kraepelin, Emil. *Lectures on Clinical Psychiatry*. Edited and Revised by Thomas Johnstone. London, 1904.
Krafft-Ebing, Richard von. *Text-Book of Insanity*. Trans. Charles Gilbert Chaddock. Philadelphia, 1905.
Kraines, Samuel Henry. *The Therapy of Neuroses and Psychoses: A Socio-Psycho-Biologic Analysis and Resynthesis*. Philadelphia, 1941.
———. *The Therapy of Neuroses and Psychoses: A Socio-Psycho-Biologic Analysis and Resynthesis*. 3rd ed. Philadelphia, 1948.
Laidlow, John, and Alan Richens, eds. *A Textbook of Epilepsy*. Edinburgh, 1976.
Lindman, Frank T., and Donald M. McIntyre, Jr., eds. *The Mentally Disabled and the Law*. Chicago, 1961.
Lockhard-Robinson, C., and Henry Maudsley. *Insanity and Crime: A Medico-Legal Commentary on the Case of George Victor Townley*. London, 1864.
MacDonald, John M. *Homicidal Threats*. Springfield, Illinois, 1968.
———. *Psychiatry and the Criminal*. 2nd ed. Springfield, Illinois, 1969.
———. *Psychiatry and the Criminal*. 3rd ed. Springfield, Illinois, 1975.
Mann, Edward C. *Insanity: Its Etiology, Diagnosis, Pathology, and Treatment, with Cases Illustrating Pathology, Morbid Histology, and Treatment*. New York, 1875.
Marc, C. C. H. *De la folie, considérée dans ses rapports avec les questions medico-judiciares*. Tome Deuxième. Paris, 1840.
Maudsley, Henry. *The Physiology and Pathology of the Mind*. London 1867.
———. *The Physiology and Pathology of the Mind*. 2nd ed. London, 1868.
———. *Responsibility in Mental Disease*. London, 1874.
May, James V. *Mental Diseases: A Public Health Problem*. Boston, 1922.
Meehl, Paul E. *Clinical versus Statistical Prediction: A Theoretical Analysis and Review of the Literature*. Minneapolis, 1954.
Menninger, Karl. *The Vital Balance: The Life Process in Mental Health and Illness*. New York, 1963.
Michu, J. L. *Discussion médico-légale, la monomanie homicide, a propos du muertre commis par Henriette Cornier*. Paris, 1826.
Nice, Richard W., ed. *Crime and Insanity*. New York, 1958.
Nicholi, Armand M., Jr., ed. *The Harvard Guide to Modern Psychiatry*. 2nd ed. Cambridge, Massachusetts, 1978.
Noyes, Arthur, P. *Modern Clinical Psychiatry*. Philadelphia, 1934.
Noyes, Arthur P., and Lawrence C. Kolb. *Modern Clinical Psychiatry*. 5th ed. Philadelphia, 1958.
Ordronaux, John. *Judicial Aspects of Insanity*. Albany, New York, 1878.
Parkman, George. *Management of Lunatics, with Illustrations of Insanity*. Boston, 1817.
———. *Proposals for Establishing a Retreat for the Insane*. Boston, 1814.
Paton, Stewart. *A Text-Book for Students and Physicians*. Philadelphia, 1905.
Penfield, Wilder, and Theodore C. Erickson. *Epilepsy and Cerebral Localization*. Springfield, Illinois, 1941.
Pfohl, Stephen J. *Predicting Dangerousness*. Lexington, Massachusetts, 1978.

Pinel, Philippe. *A Treatise on Insanity*. Trans. D. D. Davis. London, 1806.

Pitt-Lewis, George, R. Percy Smith, and J. A. Hawke. *The Insane and the Law: A Plain Guide for Medical Men, Solicitors, and Others*. London, 1895.

Prichard, James Cowles. *On the Different Forms of Insanity in Relation to Jurisprudence*. London, 1842.

————. *A Treatise on Diseases of the Nervous System. Part the First. Comprising Convulsive and Maniacal Affections*. London, 1822.

————. *A Treatise on Insanity and Other Disorders Affecting the Mind*. London, 1835.

Rappeport, Jonas R. *The Clinical Evaluation of Dangerousness in the Mentally Ill*. Washington, D.C., 1967.

Ray, Isaac. *Contributions to Mental Pathology*. Boston, 1873.

————. *A Treatise on the Medical Jurisprudence of Insanity*. Boston, 1838.

————. *A Treatise on the Medical Jurisprudence of Insanity*. 2nd ed. Boston, 1844.

————. *A Treatise on the Medical Jurisprudence of Insanity*. 5th ed. Boston, 1871.

Rees, W. L. Linford. *A Short Textbook of Psychiatry*. London, 1976.

Reynolds, J. Russell. *Epilepsy: Its Symptoms, Treatment, and Relation to Other Chronic, Convulsive Diseases*. London, 1861.

Rock, Ronald S., Marcus A. Jacobson, and Richard M. Janopaul, eds. *Hospitalization and Discharge of the Mentally Ill*. Chicago, 1968.

Rosanoff, Aaron J. *Manual of Psychiatry*. 5th ed. New York, 1905.

————. *Manual of Psychiatry*. 6th ed. New York, 1927.

————. *Manual of Psychiatry and Mental Hygiene*. 7th ed. New York, 1938.

Rush, Benjamin. *Medical Inquiries and Observations upon the Diseases of the Mind*. Philadelphia, 1812.

————. *Medical Inquiries and Observations upon the Diseases of the Mind*. 2nd ed. Philadelphia, 1818.

————. *Medical Inquiries and Observations upon the Diseases of the Mind*. 3rd ed. Philadelphia, 1827.

————. *Medical Jurisprudence*. Philadelphia, 1810.

Sampson, Marmaduke B. *Rationale of Crime, Being a Treatise on Criminal Jurisprudence, Considered in Relation to Cerebral Organization*. 2nd ed. New York, 1846.

Sands, Harry, ed. *Epilepsy: A Handbook for the Mental Health Professional*. New York, 1982.

Slaby, Andrew A., Julian Lieb, and Laurence R. Tancredi. *Psychiatric Emergencies*. 2nd ed. New York, 1981.

Smith, Stephen. *The Commitment and Detention of the Insane in the United States: Report of a Committee to the National Conference of Charities in Buffalo, [New York], June 7, 1888*. Boston, 1888.

Solomon, Philip, and Vernon D. Patch. *Handbook of Psychiatry*. 3rd ed. Los Altos, California, 1974.

Spitzka, Edward Charles. *Insanity; Its Classification, Diagnosis, and Treatment: A Manual for Students and Practitioners of Medicine*. New York, 1883.

Spratling, William Phillip. *Epilepsy and Its Treatment*. Philadelphia, 1904.

Spurzheim, Johann Cristolph. *The Anatomy of the Brain, with a General View of the Nervous System*. Trans. R. Willis. 2nd American ed. Revised by Charles H. Steadman. Boston, 1836.

————. *Observations on the Deranged Manifestations of the Mind, or Insanity*. London, 1817.

——. *Observations on the Deranged Manifestations of the Mind, or Insanity*. Boston, 1833.

——. *Phrenology, or the Doctrine of Mental Phenomena*. Boston, 1832.

Steadman, Henry J., and Joseph J. Cocozza. *Careers of the Criminally Insane*. Lexington, Massachusetts, 1974.

Stone, Alan, A. *Mental Health and Law: A System in Transition*. Rockville, Maryland, 1975.

Strecker, Edward A., and Franklin G. Ebaugh. *Practical Clinical Psychiatry*. Philadelphia, 1925.

——. *Practical Clinical Psychiatry*. 2nd ed. Philadelphia, 1928.

——. *Practical Clinical Psychiatry*. 3rd ed. Philadelphia, 1931.

——. *Practical Clinical Psychiatry*. 4th ed. Philadelphia, 1935.

——. *Practical Clinical Psychiatry*. 5th ed. Philadelphia, 1940.

Szasz, Thomas S. *Law, Liberty, and Psychiatry: An Inquiry into the Social Uses of Mental Health Practices*. New York, 1963.

——. *Psychiatric Slavery*. New York, 1977.

Taylor, Alfred S. *A Manual of Medical Jurisprudence*. London, 1844.

Taylor, James, ed. *Selected Writings of John Hughlings Jackson*. 2 vols. New York, 1958.

Thornberry, T. P., and J. E. Jacoby. *The Criminally Insane*. Chicago, 1979.

Tuke, Daniel Hack, ed. *Dictionary of Psychological Medicine*. 2 vols. London, 1892.

Upham, Thomas C. *Elements of Intellectual Philosophy*. Boston, 1827.

——. *Abridgement of Mental Philosophy*. Boston, 1861.

Wamsley, Francis H. *Outlines of Insanity*. London, 1892.

Wexter, David B. *Criminal Commitments and Dangerous Mental Patients*. Washington, D.C., 1976.

Wharton, Francis, and Moreton Stillé. *A Treatise on Medical Jurisprudence*. Philadelphia, 1855.

——. *A Treatise on Medical Jurisprudence*. 2nd ed. Philadelphia, 1860.

White, William Alanson. *Insanity and the Criminal Law*. New York, 1923.

——. *Outlines of Psychiatry*. New York, 1908.

——. *Outlines of Psychiatry*. 7th ed. Washington, D.C., 1919.

White, William Alanson, and Smith Ely Jelliffe. *Diseases of the Nervous System*. Philadelphia, 1915.

——. *Diseases of the Nervous System*. 5th ed. Philadelphia, 1929.

——, eds. *Modern Treatment of Mental and Nervous Diseases*. Philadelphia, 1913.

——. *Modern Treatment of Mental and Nervous Diseases*. 2nd ed. Philadelphia, 1929.

Winslow, Forbes B. *The Plea of Insanity in Criminal Cases*. London, 1843.

——. *On Obscure Diseases of the Brain and Disorders of the Mind*. London, 1860.

## Secondary Sources

## *Articles*

Alleridge, Patricia H., "Criminal Insanity: from Bethlem to Broadmoor," *Proceedings of the Royal Society of Medicine*, 67 (1974), 897–904.

Bridges, P. K., and J. R. Bartlett, "Psychosurgery: Yesterday and Today," *British Journal of Psychiatry*, 131 (1977) 249–60.

Burnham, John C., "Psychiatry, Psychology, and the Progressive Movement," *American Quarterly*, 12 (1960), 457–65.

Carlson, Eric T., and Norman Dain, "The Meaning of Moral Insanity," *Bulletin of the History of Medicine*, 36 (1962), 130–40.

Carlson, Eric T., and Meribeth M. Simpson, "Benjamin Rush's Medical Use of the Moral Faculty," *Bulletin of the History of Medicine*, 39 (1965), 22–33.

Dain, Norman, and Eric T. Carlson, "Moral Insanity in the United States, 1835–1866," *American Journal of Psychiatry*, 118 (1962), 795–801.

Foucault, Michael, "About the Concept of the 'Dangerous Individual' in the 19th Century Legal Psychiatry," *International Journal of Law and Psychiatry*, 1 (1978), 1–18.

Grob, Gerald N., "Samuel Woodward and the Practice of Psychiatry in Early Nineteenth-Century America," *Bulletin of the History of Medicine*, 36 (1962), 420–43.

Henry, P. F., "Psychiatric Surgery, 1935–1973: Evolution and Current Perspectives," *Canadian Psychiatric Association Journal*, 83 (1975), 157–67.

Jacyna, L. S., "Somatic Theories of the Mind and the Interests of Medicine in Britain, 1850–1879," *Medical History*, 26 (1982), 259–78.

Quen, Jacques M., "Asylum Psychiatry, Neurology, Social Work, and Mental Hygiene: An Exploratory Study in Interprofessional History," *Journal of the History of the Behavioral Sciences*, 13 (1977), 3–11.

Rosenberg, Charles, "Charles Benedict Davenport and the Beginning of Human Genetics," *Bulletin of the History of Medicine*, 35 (1961), 266–76.

Temkin, Oswei, "Gall and the Phrenological Movement," *Bulletin of the History of Medicine*, 21 (1947), 275–321.

Waldinger, Robert J., "Sleep of Reason: John P. Gray and the Challenge of Moral Insanity," *Bulletin of the History of Medicine*, 53 (1979), 163–79.

Walter, Richard D., "What Became of the Degenerate? A Brief History of the Concept," *Journal of the History of Medicine*, 11 (1956), 422–29.

## Books

Ackerknecht, Erwin A. *A Short History of Psychiatry*. Trans. Sulammith Wolfe. New York. 1959.

Bell, Leland V. *Treating the Mentally Ill from Colonial Times to the Present*. New York, 1980.

Bromberg, Walter. *Psychiatry between the Wars, 1918–1945: A Recollection*. Westport, Connecticut, 1982.

Burnham, John C. *Psychoanalysis and American Medicine, 1894–1918: Medicine, Science, and Culture*. New York, 1967.

Curti, Merle. *The Growth of American Thought*. New York, 1943.

———. *Human Nature in American Thought*. Madison, Wisconsin, 1980.

Dain, Norman. *Concepts of Insanity in the United States, 1789–1865*. New Brunswick, New Jersey, 1964.

———. *Disordered Minds: The First Century of Eastern State Hospital in Williamsburg, Virginia, 1766–1866.* Charlottesville, Virginia, 1971.

Davis, John D. *Phrenology, Fad and Science: A 19th Century American Crusade.* New Haven, Connecticut, 1955.

Deutsch, Albert. *The Mentally Ill in America: A History of Their Care and Treatment from Colonial Times.* 2nd ed. New York, 1949.

Doerner, Klaus. *Madmen and the Bourgeoisie.* Trans. Joachim Neugroschel and Jean Steinberg. Oxford, England, 1981.

Duffy, John. *The Healers: A History of American Medicine.* Chicago, 1979.

Ellenberger, Henri F. *The Discovery of the Unconscious: The History and Evolution of Dynamic Psychiatry.* New York, 1970.

Fink, Arthur E. *Causes of Crime: Biological Theories in the United States, 1880–1915.* Philadelphia, 1938.

Fox, Richard W. *So Far Disordered in Mind: Insanity in California, 1870–1930.* Berkeley, 1978.

Fullinwider, S. P. *Technicians of the Finite: The Rise and Decline of the Schizophrenic in American Thought, 1840–1960.* Westport, Connecticut, 1982.

Garrison, Fielding H. *An Introduction to the History of Medicine.* 4th ed. Philadelphia, 1929.

Grob, Gerald N. *Mental Institutions in America: Social Policy to 1875.* New York, 1973.

Gross, Samuel D., ed. *Lives of Eminent American Physicians and Surgeons of the Nineteenth Century.* Philadelphia, 1861.

Hale, Nathan G., Jr. *Freud and the Americans: The Beginning of Psychoanalysis in the United States, 1876–1917.* New York, 1971.

Haller, Mark H. *Eugenics: Hereditarian Attitudes in American Thought, 1870–1930.* New Brunswick, New Jersey, 1963.

Hare, R. D., and D. Schalling. *Psychopathic Behavior: Approaches to Research.* New York, 1975.

Hurd, Henry M., ed. *History of the Institutional Care of the Insane in the United States and Canada.* 4 vols, Baltimore, 1916.

Lief, Alfred, ed. *The Commonsense Psychiatry of Dr. Adolf Meyer.* New York, 1948.

Nye, Russel Blaine. *Society and Culture in America, 1830–1860.* New York, 1974.

Oberndorf, Clarence. *The History of Psychoanalysis in America.* New York, 1953.

Packard, Francis R. *History of Medicine in the United States.* 2 vols. New York, 1963.

Pitts, John Albert. "The Association of Medical Superintendents of American Institutions for the Insane, 1844–1892: A Case Study of Specialism in American Medicine." Ph.D. Dissertation. University of Pennsylvania, 1978.

Quen, Jacques M., and Eric T. Carlson, eds. *American Psychoanalysis: Origins and Development.* New York, 1978.

Rosenberg, Charles E. *The Trial of the Assassin Guiteau.* New York, 1968.

Schryock, Richard H. *Medicine and Society in America, 1660–1860.* New York, 1960.

Scull, Andrew T., ed. *Madhouses, Mad-Doctors and Madmen: The Social History of Psychiatry in the Victorian Era.* Philadelphia, 1981.

Sicherman, Barbara. *The Quest for Mental Health in America, 1880–1917.* New York, 1979.

Smith, Roger. *Trial by Medicine: Insanity and Responsibility in Victorian Trials*. Edinburgh, 1981.

Temkin, Oswei. *The Falling Sickness*. 2nd ed. Baltimore, 1971.

Tomes, Nancy J. *The Persuasive Institution: Thomas Story Kirkbride and the Art of Asylum Keeping*. New York, 1984.

Werlinder, Henry. *Psychopathy: A History of the Concept*. Stockholm, 1978.

# Index

## About the Author

Janet Colaizzi is a research historian
who resides in Williamsburg, Virginia.

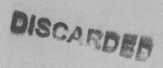